Evidence-base briefing: dementia

A compilation of secondary research evidence, guidelines and consensus statements

Claire Palmer

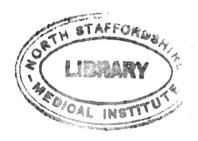

Published by Gaskell
London

British Library Cataloguing-in-Publication Data
A catalogue record for this book is available from the British Library.
ISBN 1-901242-35-8

Distributed in North America by American Psychiatric Press, Inc.
ISBN 0-88048-968-5

The Royal College of Psychiatrists is a registered charity (no. 228636).

Printed in Great Britain by Henry Ling Limited, Dorchester, Dorset.

Contents

Report compiled by: Claire Palmer, Clinical Effectiveness Projects Manager, Royal College of Psychiatrists'
Research Unit, 11 Grosvenor Crescent, London SW1X 7EE. Tel: 0171 235 2351, fax: 0171 235 2954,
e-mail: CRULondon@CompuServe.com

Preface by Roger Bullock

Reviewed by: Roger Bullock, Consultant in Old Age Psychiatry, East Wiltshire Health Care NHS Trust and
Martin Orrell, Senior Lecturer, Old Age Psychiatry, University College London

Acknowledgements: The Royal College of Psychiatrists' Research Unit is particularly grateful to Roger
Bullock and Martin Orrell for the considerable time and support they gave to this project. Publication of
this book was aided by the generous support of the East Wiltshire Health Care NHS Trust. We would also
like to thank Victoria Thomas (Clinical Effectiveness Projects Officer, Royal College of Psychiatrists' Research
Unit) for her help in preparing this EBB for publication.

Preface

Are you doing what you do well? How do you know? Do you want to see if evidence supports your belief? The answer I assume is yes or you would not have read this far. So how do you go about obtaining this evidence?

Many journals cover the subject of dementia and the papers published on the subject are rising in number exponentially. It would take the best part of working life to read everything and even longer to appraise it properly, so we have to rely on synthesised evidence and systematic summaries of published evidence. However these summaries are also increasing, so this evidence-base briefing (EBB) on dementia is an attempt to assimilate the synthesised evidence into a format which is quick and easy to use.

It is basically a list of key evidence which has been accumulated from searching centres. It does not include randomised controlled trials and is not meant to be exhaustive. It does not therefore purport to be a list of all category one evidence. Its main purpose is as a quick check-list of appraised evidence from which readers can then obtain the original documents and appraise and interpret them for their own practice.

For this reason it is broken down into accessible sections, relevant to the way we work. These sections show the area of work, a very brief summary of the evidence, the year of publication and a ranking of strength of that particular piece of evidence. The reviewer of this EBB uses a three star system to show the quality of the evidence; three being the highest. This reflects their opinion only, but is aimed at allowing readers to look at the evidence in some form of order.

There are several caveats around the use of this briefing. The evidence summary is just that – the original documents need to be read. Also, good evidence is often reviewed by many groups and so ends up listed more than once. Frequency of entry is not a reflection of importance and users of the EBB must be careful in their interpretation of the statements provided. Finally this work is, as stated, a briefing. Its aim is to point people at the evidence in order for them to appraise it and the services they offer based on it. It provides direction, not answers, and should only be used as such.

Notwithstanding, this briefing provides access to much information to support and educate. Clinical governance is becoming the order of the day. Evidence-based medicine and clinical effectiveness are two of the cornerstones of this, with care pathways and regulated standards of care becoming more frequent. National and local work will be based on the same evidence. This briefing allows people to look at what they are doing now and to develop it along with the national guidance. It can lead people to create clinical audit standards, help develop research ideas and proposals and lead to growing confidence in the knowledge and ability of those who work in the field. Decisions can be argued sensibly and information collected to add to the knowledge-base.

This is the first edition of this document. We intend to undertake a major update every two years and increase the number of sections to include other areas as more evidence appears. This is a field which is clearly continuing to expand.

This will, I hope, help to prove that you are doing what you do well and give the evidence to support it.

Roger Bullock
Consultant Psychiatrist

1. Introduction

What is an evidence-base briefing?

"Clinical information comes from two principal sources, the individual patient and research. To provide effective care, both types of information are needed." (Oxman, 1993)[1]

An evidence-base briefing (EBB) is a summarised collection of the 'evidence' (research, guidelines and national guidance) in a given topic area – in this case, dementia.

This is the first in a series of EBBs being developed by the Royal College of Psychiatrists' Research Unit. The aim of the EBB is twofold. Firstly, it aims to support clinicians in obtaining research evidence to inform their practice. Secondly, the EBB aims to promote and encourage the critical appraisal of research-based information and national guidance.

EBBs are particularly aimed at clinicians who do not have easy access to information sources such as the internet or a postgraduate library. EBBs summarise existing 'evidence' and provide details on how to access full reports – they do not make recommendations for clinical practice.

Uses of EBBs

- to generate discussion at clinical meetings
- to provide a basis for continuing professional development and education sessions
- to inform clinical audit standards
- to provide an information resource for individual practitioners or for groups
- to provide a reference/reminder resource
- to provide a basis for developing local guidelines
- to provide a basis for developing information for service users, carers and the public

While we have made every effort to ensure that the information contained in this EBB is accurate, we would recommend that it is used in conjunction with the original source documents.

Who should use this EBB?

This EBB will be useful for anyone involved in providing, managing, commissioning, using, or caring for those who use, health services for people with dementia. It is relevant to clinical and non-clinical staff, to private, voluntary and public sectors and to those working in both primary and secondary care.

How are EBBs produced?

The methods used to develop EBBs vary according to the size of the topic and the quantity, type and accessibility of the research evidence in that topic area. This dementia EBB covers a huge area of clinical practice in which there exists a large body of secondary, synthesised research. The searches for this EBB

---

1. Oxman, A., Sackett, D. & Guyatt, G. (1993) Users' guides to the medical literature: 1. How to get started. *Journal of the American Medical Association*, **270**, 2093–2095.

therefore stop at the level of secondary research and do not include searches for primary research studies. It should be noted, however, that one good quality randomised controlled trial can constitute adequate information on which to base clinical practice, and EBB users are encouraged to undertake their own searches for this level of evidence. The EBB user should also be aware that a research study may appear more than once in the EBB. For instance, the same study may be included in a systematic review, a critically appraised topic and a guideline.

The structure of this EBB

This EBB has been divided into five chapters:

1. Introduction
2. Preparing to use this EBB
3. The evidence
4. Critical appraisal tools
5. Sources of information

It is important that users of the EBB read Chapter 2 before proceeding to the evidence. Chapter 2 explains how the evidence has been compiled, the search strategy used and information on how to interpret the grading system used. Details of how to access the sources used for the EBB are provided in Chapter 5. The combination of this information should enable EBB users to update the information contained in the EBB with relative ease.

Chapter 3 comprises the main body of the EBB: the evidence. This section is a description of the evidence found using the stated search strategy. The statements are not the Royal College of Psychiatrists' guidelines for clinical practice and responsibility for interpretation of the evidence lies firmly with the EBB user. EBB users will be able to track down the source documents from the full references provided at the end of Chapter 3 and details on the source organisations are provided in Chapter 5. The evidence can be appraised using the critical appraisal tools provided in Chapter 4.

Keeping up to date

This is the key to evidence-based practice and presents a continuous struggle for all clinicians. This EBB must be viewed as a 'snap shot' of the evidence covering the time period detailed in the search strategy. The College Research Unit (CRU) strongly advises the users of this EBB to re-run the search strategy from the date given in the EBB to the present time. The CRU intends to update this EBB and undertake a major re-write every two years – resources permitting.

Participate

We would very much appreciate your feedback on this EBB – whether it is useful, how you have used it in practice, anything we have missed, ideas for developing the EBB further, suggestions for other topic areas, etc. We have provided a feedback form at the end of the publication and we very much look forward to hearing from you. We hope you find this EBB useful.

2. Preparing to use this EBB

Key to using this EBB

This chapter provides the key to using this EBB and explains how to read Chapter 3, *The evidence*.

Key to using an example page

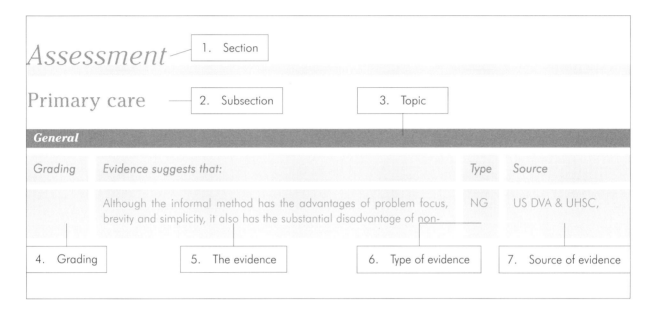

Key

1, 2 and 3.   Section, subsection and topic

The EBB is divided into subject sections to help you retrieve information quickly. The categorisation of the evidence under these headings is approximate. The statements have not been repeated in different sections. So, for example, 'Driving cessation was associated with depressive symptoms among older persons' appears under the 'Driving' section, but not under 'Depression'. Please be aware that you may need to look in several sections to find the particular topic you want.

4.   Evidence grading

Organisations producing secondary research use a variety of different grading systems. To assist the user of this EBB, the CRU has adopted a 'stars' system to allow quick comparison of evidence from different sources. Definitions for the stars have been provided in the 'Grade and strength of evidence' section.

5.   The evidence

The evidence has been compiled using the search strategy detailed on a separate sheet. Only the summary statements have been included in this EBB. Should you find evidence statements which are of interest to you, it is strongly recommended that you obtain the full reference as this often contains essential additional information.

6. Type of evidence

The evidence statements have been described as one of seven types and abbreviated as follows:

Critically appraised research summary	CARS
Economic evaluation	EE
Evidence-based guideline	EBG
Evidence-based information for purchasers	EBIP
Health technology assessment	HTA
National guidance (not necessarily evidence-based)	NG
Systematic review	SR

7. Source of evidence

A brief description of the original source of the evidence statement and year of publication, along with the abstracted source where appropriate. The full references, and details of how they might be obtained, are provided at the end of Chapter 3.

Grade and strength of evidence

Guideline and systematic review producers often provide a grade to identify the strength of evidence on which statements are based. These definitions and grades vary between organisations. This EBB therefore includes an additional scale to provide a standard guide to the evidence-base across all the sources used in the EBB.

The grading scale used in this EBB is based on that used by the Royal College of General Practitioners and is summarised below:

Grading scale used in this EBB

***   Based on at least one well-designed randomised controlled trial and recommended with substantial clinical confidence.

**   Based on well-designed cohort or case control studies and recommended with moderate clinical confidence.

*   Based on uncontrolled studies, consensus and/or extrapolated from the research. May be recommended in certain clinical situations.

Details of the original grading scales used in the EBB's source documents are provided below, along with the equivalent EBB grade. Please note: some statements in this EBB appear without an evidence grading. This is because the original documents did not identify the strength of evidence for that specific statement.

Details of the grading scales and equivalent EBB grading

Agency for Health Care Policy and Research (AHCPR)

EBB grading	AHCPR grading	Definition
***	A	Strong evidence. Evidence from studies that compare patients who have dementia with control subjects who do not have dementia but do have comorbid or interfering conditions (most difficult level of discrimination).
**	B	Suggestive evidence. The same type of evidence as in category A, but involving a smaller number of studies or a less consistent pattern of findings, or both.
*	C	Expert opinion. Evidence from clinical experience described in the literature or derived from the consensus of panel members, or both.

American Psychiatric Association (APA)

EBB grading	AHCPR grading	Definition
***	I	Recommended with substantial clinical confidence.
**	II	Recommended with moderate clinical confidence.
*	III	May be recommended on the basis of individual circumstances.

Health Care Needs Assessment (HCNA)

EBB grading	HCNA grading	Definition
***	I	Evidence obtained from at least one properly designed randomised controlled trial.
**	II-1	Evidence obtained from well-designed controlled trials without randomisation.
**	II-2	Evidence obtained from well-designed cohort or case-control analytic studies, preferably from more than one centre or research group.
**	II-3	Evidence obtained from multiple time-series with or without intervention. Dramatic results in uncontrolled experiments (e.g. the introduction of penicillin in the 1940s) could also be regarded as this type of evidence.
**	III	Opinions of respected authorities, based on clinical experience, descriptive studies or reports of expert committees.

North of England Evidence-Based Guidelines Group (EBGG)

EBB grading	EBGG grading	Definition
***	A	Directly based on category I evidence (based on well-designed randomised controlled trials, meta-analyses, or systematic reviews).
**	B	Directly based on category II evidence, or extrapolated recommendation from category I evidence. (Category II evidence is based on well-designed cohort or case control studies).
**	C	Directly based on category III evidence, or extrapolated recommendation from category I or II evidence. (Category III evidence is based on uncontrolled studies or external consensus).
**	D	Based on the group's clinical opinion.

Quality Standards Subcommittee of the American Academy of Neurology (AAN)

EBB grading	AAN grading	Definition
***	Standards	Generally accepted principles for patient management that reflect a high degree of clinical certainty (i.e. based on class I evidence or, when circumstances preclude randomised clinical trials, overwhelming evidence from class II studies that directly addresses the question at hand or from decision analysis that directly addresses all the issues). (Class I is evidence provided by one or more well-designed randomised controlled clinical trials; class II is evidence provided by one or more well-designed clinical studies such as case-control studies, cohort studies, and so forth).
**	Guidelines	Recommendations for patient management that may identify a particular strategy or range of management strategies and that reflect moderate clinical certainty (i.e. based on class II evidence that directly addresses the issue, decision analysis that directly addresses the issue, or strong consensus of class III evidence). (Class III is evidence provided by expert opinion, non-randomised historical controls, or one or more case reports).
*	Practice opinions/ guidelines	Other strategies for patient management for which there is unclear clinical certainty (i.e. based on inconclusive or conflicting evidence or opinion). Practice options in certain clinical situations may be considered medically indicated.
–	Practice parameters	Results, in the form of one or more specific recommendations, from a scientifically-based analysis of a specific clinical problem.

Scottish Intercollegiate Guidelines Network (SIGN)

EBB grading	SIGN	Definition
***	A	Required: at least one randomised controlled trial as part of the body of literature of overall good quality and consistency addressing specific recommendation.
**	B	Required: availability of well conducted clinical studies but no randomised clinical trials on the topic or recommendation.
*	C	Required: evidence obtained from expert committee reports or opinions and/or clinical experiences of respected authorities.

US Preventive Services Task Force (US PSTF)

EBB grading	US PSTF grading	Definition
***	A	Indicates that there is good evidence to support the recommendation that the condition be specifically considered in a periodic health examination.
**	B	Indicates that there is fair evidence to support the recommendation that the condition be specifically considered.
*	C	Indicates that there is insufficient evidence to support the recommendation that the condition be specifically considered.
-	D	Indicates that there is fair evidence to support the recommendation that the condition be excluded from consideration in a periodic health examination.
-	E	Indicates that there is good evidence to support the recommendation that the condition be excluded from consideration in a periodic health examination.

Search strategy

The search strategy describes the sources searched for information to include in this EBB. The keywords used in the searching were: dementia and Alzheimer's. The authors do not accept responsibility for any information which has been missed during the searching. Further details on these sources are provided in Chapter 5.

Evidence	Source	From	To
All types	Oxamweb at the Centre for Evidence-Based Mental Health	All	Aug 1998
Guideline	AHCPR	All	July 1998
	SIGN	All	July 1998
	APA	All	Aug 1998
	Royal College of Psychiatrists library and CD ROM: ClinPsyc	1988	June 1998
	Medline	1991	Sept 1998
	In-house collection	All	Sept 1998
	RCPsych Research Unit's *Guidelines Bibliography*	All	Aug 1998
	Guideline database	All	July 1998
Systematic reviews	Cochrane Library, including the Database of Abstracts of Reviews of Effectivness (DARE)	Issue 3	July 1998
	NHS Centre for Reviews and Dissemination (NHS CRD) publications, e.g. *Effective Health Care* bulletins and *Effectiveness Matters*	All	July 1998
Health technology assessments	Health Technology Assessment Database (at CRD)	All	July 1998
	Development and Evaluation Committee (DEC) reports	All	July 1998
Economic evaluations	National Economic Evaluation Database (NEED) (at CRD)	All	July 1998
Information for patients	Centre for Health Information Quality (CHiQ)	All	July 1998

Evidence	Source	From	To
Outcomes	UK Clearing House on Health Outcomes	All	July 1998
Evidence-based information for patients	Trent Working Group	All	July 1998
	Scottish Health Purchasing Information Centre	All	July 1998
	Evidence-based purchasing	All	July 1998
	Health Evidence bulletins – Wales	All	July 1998
Critically-appraised research summaries	American College of Physicians	1991	July 1998
	Evidence-Based Medicine	1995	July 1998
	Evidence-Based Mental Health	Jan 1998	July 1998
	Evidence-Based Nursing	Jan 1998	July 1998
	Evidence-Based Practice Patient-Oriented Evidence that Matters (POEMs)	All	July 1998
	Bandolier	All	July 1998
Critically appraised research summaries	Aggressive Research Intelligence Facility (ARIF)	All	July 1998
	Critically Appraised Topic (CAT) Bank	All	July 1998
	Therapeutics Initiative	All	July 1998
	The National Preferred Medicines Centre Inc (PreMec)	All	July 1998
Other	Standing Medical Advisory Committee	All	July 1998
	Joseph Rowntree Foundation	All	Aug 1998
	Department of Health: Circulars on the Internet (COIN)	All	Aug 1998
	Relevant voluntary sector organisations	All	Sept 1998

Abbreviations

ACCG	*Abstracts of Clinical Care Guidelines*
ACP	American College of Physicians
AHCPR	Agency for Health Care Policy Research
APA	American Psychiatric Association
CAT	Critically Appraised Topic
CEBM	Centre for Evidence-Based Medicine
CHSR	Centre for Health Studies Research (and Department of Primary Care)
DARE	Database of Abstracts of Reviews of Effectiveness
EBM	*Evidence-Based Medicine*
EBMH	*Evidence-Based Mental Health*
EBN	*Evidence-Based Nursing*
NEED	NHS Economic Evaluation Database
NHS CRD	NHS Centre for Reviews and Dissemination
POEM	Patient-Oriented Evidence that Matters
RCPsych	Royal College of Psychiatrists
RCGP	Royal College of General Practitioners
SIGN	Scottish Intercollegiate Guidelines Network
US DVA & UHSC	US Department of Veteran Affairs and University Health System Consortium

3. The evidence

Introduction

Chapter 2, *Preparing to use this EBB*, should be read before proceeding to this section. This provides information on the grading system, the type and source of evidence, how the evidence has been compiled and how it should be used.

Chapter 3 has been organised to reflect clinical practice to some extent. It begins, therefore, with assessment and then progresses through quality of life, issues related to carers and families, clinical management, psychosocial and medication interventions and then particular issues related to people with learning disabilities who have dementia. The section ends with a full list of references.

Assessment

Primary care

General

Grading	Evidence suggests that:	Type	Source
	Although the informal method has the advantages of problem focus, brevity and simplicity, it also has the substantial disadvantage of non-standardisation and dependence on the examiner's expertise. Clinicians using it should add tests of attention, memory, language, visuospatial status and executive functions.	NG	US DVA & UHSC, 1997
	Primary care practitioners have two options for starting the evaluation: an informal clinical mental status examination (practical questions addressed to the patient to test orientation) or a structured mental status assessment questionnaire.	NG	As above

When to refer to a specialist

Grading	Evidence suggests that:	Type	Source
*	Referral for neuropsychological, neurological, or psychiatric evaluation should be made if mixed results – abnormal findings on the functional assessment with normal mental status performance or vice versa – are obtained.	EBG	AHCPR, 1996
	The specialist old age psychiatry service routinely deals with all aspects, stages and varieties of psychiatric disorder arising in old age. Thereby it is skilled and experienced in recognising not only dementia, but also psychiatric disorder which may mimic or complicate it. It also deals with all stages of dementia, providing continuing care for severe cases, and accumulates expertise (both recognition and management skills) with the full range of problems which can develop over time.	NG	RCPsych, 1995

Assessment

When to refer to a specialist (continued)

Grading	Evidence suggests that:	Type	Source
	If the initial assessment (including history, functional evaluation, psychiatric assessment, mental status examination, neurological/physical examination, care-giver assessment) does not clearly determine the presence of a dementia syndrome, the patient may be referred for speciality evaluation, such as: neuropsychological assessment to distinguish dementia from normal ageing; psychiatric and/or neuro-psychological consultation to distinguish dementia from depression; or medical assessment to differentiate delirium from dementia.	NG	US DVA & UHSC, 1997
	Further assessment may be required to clarify the diagnosis, to explore aggravating factors more fully or to elucidate aetiology. Admission to the district general hospital acute assessment ward (a core service element) may be necessary but usually this additional assessment can be accomplished in the day hospital (a core service element), in an out-patient clinic, or at home. Striving to enable the patient to remain at home at the highest possible level of functioning is the emphasis throughout.	NG	RCPsych, 1995

Home assessment

Grading	Evidence suggests that:	Type	Source
	Home assessment should be part of the routine initial assessment offered for all new cases, although initial assessment of those in other settings would not be delayed on this basis, and with some cases (e.g. routine assessment in the memory clinic) it may be deemed unnecessary or inappropriate. This assessment should be made by a senior doctor of the service. Also, all members of the multi-disciplinary team should be available as appropriate for involvement in such assessments. In some services other team members make at least the initial home assessment, but this should always be under the supervision of the specialist.	NG	RCPsych, 1995

Primary care investigations

Grading	Evidence suggests that:	Type	Source
	Possible investigations by general practitioners include: • full blood count • B12 • folate • thyroid-stimulating hormone • gamma-glutamyl transferase • syphilis serology • midstream urine • chest X-ray	NG	Haines & Katona, 1992 (RCGP)

History and presentation

General

Grading	Evidence suggests that:	Type	Source
***	The core of the treatment of patients with dementia is psychiatric management, which must be based on a solid alliance with the patient and family and thorough psychiatric, neurological and general medical evaluations of the nature and cause of the cognitive deficits and associated non-cognitive symptoms.	EBG	APA, 1997
**	Health care professionals should be aware of the increased incidence and prevalence of dementia with increasing age.	EBG	CHSR, 1998
**	An initial clinical assessment that combines multiple and varied sources of information, is recommended to evaluate patients with suspected dementia.	EBG	AHCPR, 1996
*	Assessment, both medical and social, is obviously needed but there is no guide as to how intensive a process it should be. Medical assessment can be carried out in many different ways ranging from a brief examination and review in the GP surgery to a four week in-patient stay. The relative effectiveness of each of these methods for different categories of patients has not been assessed.	EBIP	Melzer et al, 1994
	Where possible, the assessment should be carried out by an inter-disciplinary team in which each component is carried out by the team member most qualified to administer that particular portion. • One member of the team should be responsible for coordinating the assessment. • The members of the team should meet with the care-givers to communicate the findings of the assessment and discuss how to adapt care and access services in response to identified needs and abilities.	NG	Alzheimer Society of Canada, 1992
	A full assessment should lead to the creation of an individual 'care package' regularly reviewed to remain sensitive to changing needs.	NG	Haines & Katona, 1992 (RCGP)

New referrals

Grading	Evidence suggests that:	Type	Source
	Assessment of all referrals accepted by the service should be under the supervision of the consultant (or medical deputy). Best practice is for all such new cases to be seen by a medical member of the team and resources should allow this. All medical referrals should be seen by a doctor of the service.	NG	RCPsych, 1995

Assessment

Symptoms

Grading	Evidence suggests that:	Type	Source
**	Health care professionals should be aware that complaints of subjective memory impairment are not a good indicator of dementia. A history of loss of function is more indicative than memory impairment.	EBG	CHSR, 1998
**	Individuals who should be evaluated for evidence of dementia include: those with memory or other cognitive complaints with or without functional impairment; elderly patients in whom there is a question of incompetency; patients with depression or anxiety with cognitive complaints; and patients who arouse physician suspicion of cognitive impairment during their interview despite the absence of complaints.	EBG	American Academy of Neurology, 1994
*	The symptoms possibly indicating dementia listed below provide clues to the health care provider for recognition and initial assessment of dementia. Does the person have increased difficulty with any of these activities?<ul><li>Learning and retaining new information; is repetitive: has trouble remembering recent conversations, events, appointments; frequently misplaces objects.</li><li>Handling complex tasks: has trouble following a complex train of thought or performing tasks that require many steps such as balancing a cheque-book or cooking a meal.</li><li>Reasoning ability: is unable to respond with a reasonable plan to problems at work or home, such as knowing what to do if the bathroom is flooded; shows uncharacteristic disregard for rules of social conduct.</li><li>Spatial ability and orientation; has trouble driving, organising objects around the house, finding his or her way around familiar places.</li><li>Language: has increasing difficulty with finding the words to express what he or she wants to say and with following conversations.</li><li>Behaviour: appears more passive and less responsive; is more irritable than usual; is more suspicious than usual; misinterprets visual or auditory stimuli.</li></ul>	EBG	AHCPR, 1996

Safety

Grading	Evidence suggests that:	Type	Source
***	Safety measures include: evaluation of suicidality and the potential for violence; recommendations regarding adequate supervision, preventing falls and limiting the hazards of wandering; vigilance regarding neglect or abuse; and restrictions on driving and use of other dangerous equipment.	EBG	APA, 1997
	The assessment should address the safety and security of the person with Alzheimer's disease and of their care-givers.<ul><li>The assessment should address the care-givers' ability to provide the type of care required by the individual with Alzheimer's disease.</li><li>The assessment should describe the quality and adequacy of the social support systems.</li><li>The assessment should identify the need for formal community services, such as a day programme, to collaborate with the informal social support network.</li></ul>	NG	Alzheimer Society of Canada, 1992

Safety (continued)

Grading	Evidence suggests that:	Type	Source
	Wandering is common; an effort should be made to understand the cause, such as changes in the environment.	NG	ACCG, 1997b (from Post & Whitehouse, 1995)

Aggressive behaviour

Grading	Evidence suggests that:	Type	Source
	There is a relationship between delusions and aggressive behaviour. Aggressive behaviour should be assessed with this in mind.	EBG	CHSR, 1998

Difficulty gaining patient cooperation

Grading	Evidence suggests that:	Type	Source
	Practical difficulties or lack of cooperation by the patient may prevent the preferred plan of investigation, aimed both at aetiological and aggravating factors. It will be unusual for use of compulsion via mental health legislation to appear justifiable to override such difficulty with investigation in the assessment of dementia.	EBG	RCPsych, 1995

Social

Grading	Evidence suggests that:	Type	Source
	The assessment should address the social circumstances of the person with Alzheimer's disease and of their care-givers. • The assessment should address the care-givers' ability to provide the type of care required by the individual with Alzheimer's disease. • The assessment should describe the quality and adequacy of the social support systems. • The assessment should identify the need for formal community services, such as a day program, to collaborate with the informal social support network.	EBG	Alzheimer Society of Canada, 1992

History taking

Grading	Evidence suggests that:	Type	Source
**	Health care professionals should be aware of the diminution of insight as dementia progresses, making the patient's history less reliable.	EBG	CHSR, 1998
*	A focused history is critical in the assessment of dementia. The history should include relevant medical, family, social, cultural and medication history (including alcohol use), as well as a detailed description of the chief complaint.	EBG	AHCPR, 1996

Assessment

Using informants

Grading	Evidence suggests that:	Type	Source
**	Because of the potential unreliability of the patient's history, a history of memory problems should be sought from a carer as well as the patient when assessing a person with cognitive impairment.	EBG	CHSR, 1998
*	The history should be obtained from the patient and a reliable informant.	EBG	AHCPR, 1996
✓	Documentation of a full history from an informant is essential to clarify the onset and course of the cognitive impairment, the degree of functional incapacity (e.g. continence, dressing, feeding, ability to handle financial affairs) and the current network of informal and statutory support. Areas of carer stress and specific deficiencies in care can also be identified. Examination of the mental state requires a high index of suspicion for depression and for acute organic states as well as the need to look out for dysphasias, dyspraxias and agnosias.	NG	Haines & Katona, 1992 (RCGP)
✓	Collateral (family/carer) history should be sought as part of the assessment process in all cases and is usually obtained from the family/carer individual most closely involved. This will both elaborate the clinical history and help specify the problems to be tackled. Discussion and planning for future care is also begun at this stage.	NG	RCPsych, 1995

Assessment process

General

Grading	Evidence suggests that:	Type	Source
***	The neurological history and examination (including mental status examination) are essential components of the diagnostic work-up – and may reveal clues to the aetiology of the patient's dementia.	EBG	American Academy of Neurology, 1994
*	Health care professionals should be sensitive to the possible coexistence of dementia and other psychiatric symptomatology (delusions and/or hallucinations), usually persecutory in nature and simple in type.	EBG	CHSR, 1998
	Each individual should receive a comprehensive assessment to identify his or her needs, strengths and abilities, weaknesses and personal characteristics. • The assessment should evaluate the individual's cognitive function, physical, mental, emotional and spiritual status, social function, and ability to carry out activities of daily living. • A personal history should also be included as part of the assessment. • The assessment should be carried out in a familiar environment in which the individual feels comfortable. • Results of recently completed assessments and diagnostic tests should be incorporated into the current assessment to reduce duplication of effort and stress for the individual being assessed.	NG	Alzheimer Society of Canada, 1992

General (continued)

Grading	Evidence suggests that:	Type	Source
	At the final stage of the assessment the clinician considers a group of disorders characterised by the absence of elementary neurological abnormalities, normal imaging or imaging that reveals only cerebral atrophy, and normal laboratory results. These include: Alzheimer's disease (by far the most common); frontotemporal dementias; Lewy body dementia. The pattern of cognitive and behavioural changes may help distinguish between these. Accurate differential diagnosis depends on integrating psychiatric assessment with findings on the mental status exam and neuropsychological testing. The current diagnostic accuracy for Alzheimer's disease when research diagnostic criteria are applied, is 85% to 90%.	NG	US DVA & UHSC, 1997

Techniques/methods

Grading	Evidence suggests that:	Type	Source
*	Most neurologists gather information regarding cognitive decline, presence of depression, evidence of vascular disease and social and occupational functioning by history. Many of these elements have been incorporated into instruments that, especially in research settings, may assist the clinician in diagnosis.	EBG	American Academy of Neurology, 1994
*	The techniques used to assess level of arousal, attention, orientation, recent and remote memory, language, praxis, visuospatial function, calculations and judgement, are at the discretion of the individual physician.	EBG	As above

Mental status tests

Grading	Evidence suggests that:	Type	Source
***	Currently, no single mental status test is clearly superior, and any of the tests recommended in the guidelines may be used. Tests recommended in the guidelines are: the Mini-Mental State Examination (MMSE; Folstein et al, 1975), the Blessed Information–Memory Concentration Test (Katzman et al, 1983), the Blessed Orientation–Memory Concentration Test (Katzman et al, 1983) and the Short Test of Mental Status (Kokmen et al, 1987).	EBG	AHCPR, 1996
** *	Health care professionals should consider the use of the following instruments as tools in helping to identify cognitive impairment: • the MMSE • the clock drawing test • an instrument for assessing activities of daily living, e.g. Clifton Assessment Procedures for the Elderly (Pattie & Gilleard, 1975); and • Abbreviated Mental Test Score (Hodkinson, 1972)	EBG	CHSR, 1998
**	Cognitive or mental status testing should include assessment of level of arousal, attention, orientation, recent and remote memory, language, praxis, visuospatial function, calculations and judgement.		American Academy of Neurology, 1994

Assessment

Mental status tests (continued)

Grading	Evidence suggests that:	Type	Source
**	Confounding factors such as age, educational level and cultural influences should be assessed and considered in the interpretation of mental status test scores.	EBG	AHCPR, 1996
**	Factors such as visual impairment, sensory impairment and physical disability should be assessed and considered in the selection of mental status tests.	EBG	As above
*	Further clinical evaluation should be conducted if abnormal findings are obtained for both mental status and functional status tests.	EBG	As above
*	If both mental and functional status tests are normal and no other concerns have been raised in the clinical assessment, reassurance by the treating health professional is recommended, together with a suggestion for reassessment in 6–12 months. If concerns persist despite normal mental status and functional assessment results, referral for a second opinion or further clinical evaluation is appropriate.	EBG	As above
*	A variety of useful and well-validated clinical criteria are available for diagnosis of Alzheimer's disease.	EBG	American Academy of Neurology, 1994
*	Neuropsychological evaluation is recommended in the following circumstances: (a) When the mental status test, conducted as part of an initial assessment for possible dementia, is abnormal, but the functional assessment is normal. (b) When a family member expresses concern or there is suspicion about dementia, the results of mental status tests are within the normal range, and the patient has (i) more than a high school education or (ii) an occupation that indicates high premorbid intelligence. (c) When mental status test results indicate cognitive impairment and the patient: (i) has low formal education (ii) shows evidence of long-term low intelligence (more than 10 years) (iii) does not have adequate command of English for the test (iv) is of minority racial or ethnic background (v) is impaired in only one area of cognitive functioning on mental status tests (vi) does not have evidence of cognitive impairment of more than six months; or (vii) does not show functional impairments.	EBG	AHCPR, 1996
	The guideline recommends adopting a brief, standardised mental status questionnaire with operationalised criteria for defining an abnormal performance, suggesting either the MMSE, the Blessed Information–Memory Concentration Test, the Blessed Orientation–Memory Concentration Test, or the Short Test of Mental Status.	NG	US DVA & UHSC, 1997
	The MMSE and Informant Questionnaire on Cognitive Decline were efficient screening tests for dementia.	CARS	*EBM*, 1997a (from Mulligan *et al*, 1997)
	A documented clinical examination aims to elucidate any mental state abnormalities present, and particularly elaborates deficits of cognitive function. Standardised mental test questions for cognitive function may be included (e.g. MMSE, Abbreviated Mental Test Score, or the Clifton Assessment Procedures for the Elderly). This is linked to the available history of the development of the problem and observations on any immediately evident physical illness.	NG	RCPsych, 1995

Functional status tests

Grading	Evidence suggests that:	Type	Source
***	The Functional Activities Questionnaire (Pfeffer *et al*, 1982) is useful in the initial assessment for functional impairment.	EBG	AHCPR, 1996

Neurophysical evaluation

Grading	Evidence suggests that:	Type	Source
*	Although not generally necessary, neuropsychological testing may be helpful in: (a) demonstrating cognitive impairment in individuals whose initial evaluation is borderline or suspicious; (b) distinguishing depression from dementia; (c) determining competency for legal purposes; and (d) assisting in the evaluation of early dementia, particularly when major decisions need to be made with regard to a patient's job (e.g. disability determination) or other personal affairs.	EBG	American Academy of Neurology, 1994

Physical examination

Grading	Evidence suggests that:	Type	Source
	Associated physical illness commonly leads to worsened functioning, behaviour or dependency which can be improved with successful specific treatment. Similarly, physical illness in the carer, social/family/ psychological stresses, or other factors affecting either the patient or the carer, can produce a potentially reversible exacerbation. Initial assessment (and, often necessary, further assessment) identifies and documents such factors.	NG	RCPsych, 1995
	It is essential that an adequate physical examination, aimed at detecting indications of aetiology or of aggravating factors, is undertaken in the assessment process. This will usually be conducted by the GP (or other referring doctor) but may be performed (or added to) by the specialist team. Certainly, they will wish to include the results of such an examination in their assessment.	NG	RCPsych, 1995

Diagnostic issues

Possible delirium and/or depression

Grading	Evidence suggests that:	Type	Source
***	Patients with dementia and depression may best be differentiated by a memory task that uses delayed retrieval with distraction. (Centre for Reviews and Dissemination commentary on meta-analysis provided. It is recommended that this is consulted before acting upon this evidence).	SR	DARE; NHS CRD, 1998b (from Lachner & Engel, 1994)
***	Patients with depression should be carefully evaluated for suicide potential.	EBG	APA, 1997
**	The clinician should seek evidence for delirium and depression during the initial clinical assessment.	EBG	AHCPR, 1996

Assessment

Possible delirium and/or depression (continued)

Grading	Evidence suggests that:	Type	Source
	It is important to distinguish dementia from delirium (acute confusional state) and depression. • Delirium usually indicates an underlying physical cause such as infection of drug toxicity. The history is usually acute, with deterioration over a few days or weeks, and it may of course be superimposed on pre-existing dementia. The characteristic presenting feature is of a patient with a fluctuating level of consciousness. Other features which suggest delirium rather than dementia include hallucinations and intense fearfulness. Dementia does not in itself cause clouding of consciousness. • Depression should be considered particularly where there is a relatively short history (weeks or months) and in patients who are withdrawn or apathetic and who appear indifferent to the assessment process. Depression is important to diagnose because of the likelihood of response to treatment. It may coexist with dementia in its early stages. In this case there may be a fairly clear onset of cognitive impairment rather than an insidious onset over a long period, which is a characteristic of Alzheimer's disease alone.	NG	Haines & Katona, 1992 (RCGP)
	Diagnosis of the dementia syndrome (or of other illness) is made on the basis of the clinical information provided by the specialist medical staff of the team, carefully considering other possibilities such as delirium or depressive illness with pseudo-dementia.	NG	RCPsych, 1995

Possible dementia with Lewy bodies

Grading	Evidence suggests that:	Type	Source
**	Health care professionals should be aware of the importance of differentially diagnosing dementia with Lewy Bodies because of the high risk of increased morbidity and mortality with neuroleptic agents in these patients.	EBG	CHSR, 1998

Vascular dementia

Grading	Evidence suggests that:	Type	Source
***	Health care professionals should be aware that stroke is a significant risk factor in the development of vascular dementia.	EBG	CHSR, 1998
*	A diagnosis of vascular dementia is supported by: (a) the sudden onset of dysfunction in one or more cognitive domains; (b) a stepwise deteriorating course; (c) focal neurological signs, including weakness of an extremity, exaggeration of deep tendon reflexes, extensor plantar responses and gait abnormalities; (d) history or neuroimaging evidence of previous strokes; and (e) evidence of stroke risk factors and systemic vascular disease. These clinical features have been incorporated into a number of different clinical criteria or 'ischemic' scores.	EBG	American Academy of Neurology, 1994

No obvious cause for dementia

Grading	Evidence suggests that:	Type	Source
	If no obvious cause of a patient's dementia can be found, a diagnostic evaluation should be initiated, combining the history and examinations with laboratory studies and possibly including more advanced studies such as neuroimaging, neuropsychological assessment, functional neuroimaging, electrophysiological studies and specialised laboratory tests. These steps are followed by assessment for a motor system disorder, such as Parkinsonian syndromes with dementia, and then by assessment for a dementia syndrome of depression.	NG	US DVA & UHSC, 1997

Unable to make a diagnosis

Grading	Evidence suggests that:	Type	Source
*	Some patients may not meet criteria for dementia even though they or their families are concerned about changes in intellectual functioning. This group may include well-educated, high-functioning individuals, patients with psychiatric problems (e.g. depression or anxiety) and patients with early or very mild dementia who may be considered to be at risk for dementia. These patients should be encouraged to return for re-evaluation, since observation over time, often 6–12 months, may help to document cognitive decline. For these patients, neuropsychological testing is often valuable to detect subtle cognitive difficulties.	EBG	American Academy of Neurology, 1994
	Patients for whom no diagnosis can be assigned confidently should be followed and reassessed periodically, during which time clinicians can treat emergent behavioural problems, work with the care-givers as the dementia progresses and consult with experts in other disciplines as needed.	NG	US DVA & UHSC, 1997
	Ongoing assessments should monitor changes in the individual and his or her circumstances. • Reassessments should be carried out at least every six months and more frequently if physical, mental or behavioural changes in the individual suggest the care plan may need to be revised. • A reassessment should deal only with those areas in which additional information will contribute to improved care.	NG	Alzheimer Society of Canada, 1992

Depression

Grading	Evidence suggests that:	Type	Source
*	Consider relevant risk factors for depressive illness such as personal or family history of depression or recent adverse events such as bereavement or relocation.	EBG	CHSR, 1998
*	The history from patients assessed for depression should be gathered from both the patients and their carers.	EBG	As above

Assessment

Depression (continued)

Grading	Evidence suggests that:	Type	Source
*	Health care professionals should have a high index of suspicion for diagnosing depression in patients with dementia at any stage in the dementia process.	EBG	CHSR, 1998
	Depression is common in patients with dementia.	EBG	APA, 1997

Investigations

General

Grading	Evidence suggests that:	Type	Source
	In all cases careful consideration should be given, in the light of the clinical evidence, to what investigation is appropriate and could be achieved. In nearly all cases some investigation has been or can be achieved, by either the secondary or the primary care teams, and any such opportunity should be exploited. Management arrangements should aim to ensure that results of examinations or tests are available to the specialist team. With present knowledge, most investigation during life serves mainly to elucidate and eliminate aggravating factors. It is unusual for potentially reversible causes of dementia to be revealed, although it is most important to look for them, and in time matters will change.	NG	RCPsych, 1995

Routine investigations

Grading	Evidence suggests that:	Type	Source
**	The detailed work-up depends on the suspected diagnosis, but generally should include the following tests: complete blood cell count, serum electrolytes (including calcium), glucose, blood urea nitrogen/creatinine, liver function tests, thyroid function tests (free thyroid index and thyroid-stimulating hormone), serum vitamin B12 level, and syphilis serology. Other tests may be helpful but are not recommended as routine studies. These include: sedimentation rate, serum folate level, HIV testing, chest X-ray, urinalysis, 24-hour urine collection for heavy metals, toxicology screen, neuroimaging study (CT or MRI), neuropsychological testing, lumbar puncture, electroencephalography, positron emission tomography, and single-photon emission computed tomography.	EBG	American Academy of Neurology, 1994
**	Diagnostic tests are necessary in the differential diagnosis of dementia to rule out metabolic and structural causes.	EBG	As above
	There is insufficient firm evidence yet to allow authoritative recommend-ation of a definitive list of investigations which should always be performed.	NG	RCPsych, 1995

Neuroimaging

Grading	Evidence suggests that:	Type	Source
*	EEG is not recommended as a routine study but may assist in distinguishing depression or delirium from dementia and in evaluating for suspected encephalitis, Creutzfeldt–Jakob disease, metabolic encephalopathy or seizures.	EBG	American Academy of Neurology, 1994
	A CT scan is helpful in confirming normal pressure hydrocephalus and contributes to the distinction between Alzheimer's disease and multi-infarct dementia as well as clearly showing subdural haematomas. Except where normal pressure hydrocephalus or subdural haematoma is suspected on clinical grounds, the CT scan is unlikely to alter management and, in view of its expense, is not routinely indicated in patients aged over 75 years in whom the clinical picture is unequivocally of a dementia.	NG	Haines & Katona, 1992 (RCGP)

Lumbar puncture

Grading	Evidence suggests that:	Type	Source
**	Lumbar puncture should be performed (assuming there are no contra-indications) when any of the following is present: • metastatic cancer • suspicion of central nervous system infection • reactive serum syphilis serology • hydrocephalus • dementia in a person younger than 55 years of age • a rapidly progressive or unusual dementia • immunosuppression • suspicion of central nervous system vasculitis, particularly in patients with connective tissue diseases	EBG	American Academy of Neurology, 1994
	Lumbar puncture is not recommended as a routine study in the evaluation of dementia.	EBG	As above

Assessment

27

Quality of life

General			
Grading	**Evidence suggests that:**	**Type**	**Source**
	This study found the following: • Between 68 and 73% of the sample were happy with their overall quality of life. • Poor and worsening levels of satisfaction were most closely associated with some worsening ability to perform everyday tasks and with declining health status. • Anxiety and depression were consistently associated with poor or deteriorating levels of ability to perform routine tasks. Improvements in these abilities and in physical health led to improvements in mental health. • In the sample of people aged 85 years and over, after allowing for differences in health, men with few social contacts had a higher risk of death than others, while women who belonged to social clubs had a better chance of living longer. • The earlier detection of treatable health problems (eyesight, hearing, feet, arthritis, anxiety and depression) might lead to reductions in depression and anxiety and an increase in life satisfaction for very elderly people. (For complete set of results please see full report).	SRR	Bowling *et al*, 1997
	'Low level' preventive services, like help with housework, gardening, laundry and home maintenance and repairs, both enhance quality of life for older people and help them maintain their independence. The study found that keeping a well-maintained house was central to many older people's sense of well-being and of being part of society, as well as to their confidence about coping at home.	SRR	As above
	Care-givers need to learn what makes the person with dementia feel happy.	NG	*ACCG, 1997b* (from Post & Whitehouse, 1995)
	Quality of life in people with dementia is difficult to assess because it includes a subjective element. Those who are cognitively intact must avoid assertions that ignore this element.	NG	As above

Screening/prevention

General

Grading	Evidence suggests that:	Type	Source
**	Population screening for dementia in those over 65 years of age is not recommended. A case-finding approach is recommended.	EBG	CHSR, 1998
*	There is insufficient evidence to recommend for or against routine screening for dementia with standardised instruments in asymptomatic persons. Clinicians should remain alert for possible signs of declining cognitive function in older patients and evaluate mental status in patients who have problems performing daily activities. Clinicians should periodically ask patients about their functional status at home and at work, and they should remain alert to changes in performance with age. When possible, information about daily activities should be solicited from family members or other persons. Brief tests such as the Mini-Mental State Examination (Folstein *et al*, 1975) should be used to assess cognitive function in patients in whom the suspicion of dementia is raised by restrictions in daily activities, concerns of family members and other evidence of worsening function (e.g. trouble with finances, medications, transportation). Possible effects of education and cultural differences should be considered when interpreting results of cognitive tests. The diagnosis of dementia should not be based on results of screening tests alone. Patients suspected of having dementia should be examined for other causes of changing mental status, including depression, delirium, medication effects and coexisting medical illness.	EBG	US Preventive Services Task Force, 1996
*	There is no evidence that population screening or early recognition is of benefit. Population screening for dementia has not been evaluated in the UK. Although frequently advocated, there is no evidence that early recognition alters the natural history of the disease or that it benefits the patient or the carer. Early recognition may raise a problem as it is difficult to distinguish mild cognitive impairment from the natural ageing process. Providing a label of dementia in the early stages may cause psychological distress and disrupt a caring relationship. The introduction of annual health checks for the over-75s and three-yearly checks for the under-75s introduced with the 1990 GP contract are as yet unevaluated in terms of screening and early recognition of dementia.	EBIP	Melzer *et al*, 1994
	There is no evidence for successful prevention of dementia of the Alzheimer's type. Programmes related to healthy lifestyle, reduction in blood pressure and avoidance of head injury which may be of value in non-Alzheimer's type dementia have been evaluated with other end-points in mind (e.g. cardiovascular disease events and death). Genetic counselling has a role to play in prevention of dementias associated with, for example, Down's syndrome and Huntington's chorea).	EBIP	As above
	Test characteristics and pretest probability of disease need to be considered in screening for dementia.	CARS	*ACP Journal Club*, 1991*b* (from Sui, 1991)

Genetic testing

Grading	Evidence suggests that:	Type	Source
	Genetic testing of symptomatic individuals with suspected early-onset autosomal dominant Alzheimer's disease can now be accomplished but, as for predictive testing, diagnostic genetic test results need to be cautiously interpreted. Since the experts cannot agree, the work group suggests that primary care physicians not yet consider APOE part of the diagnostic evaluation of dementia.	NG	*ACCG, 1997a (from Post et al, 1997)*
	When APOE testing is done in the course of a medically-indicated evaluation of serum lipid profiles for managing cardiovascular disease, the patients should be prospectively informed of the supplemental information relating to Alzheimer's disease and should be advised that: (a) the testing unavoidably determines whether a gene related to Alzheimer's disease is present; (b) there may be implications for recording these data in the medical record; and (c) they have the option to have a discussion about the Alzheimer's disease implications of this testing.	NG	As above
	The major concern in APOE genetic testing is unnecessary anxiety, which could lead to precipitous decisions based on the misinterpretation of risk.	NG	As above
	Predictive use of APOE testing in symptomatic individuals is not recommended at this time.	NG	As above
	Genetic testing for mutations associated with an increased risk for Alzheimer's disease, Huntington's disease or spinocerebellar degenerations may be useful, particularly for those with an unusual presentation of dementia or for whom a diagnosis is needed to permit therapy with agents limited to Alzheimer's disease. Individuals interested in genetic testing should seek genetic counselling before the testing is ordered and after the results are obtained.	NG	As above
	Genetic counselling is an integral component of predictive testing programmes, which should: (a) clarify the potential benefits and burdens of testing outcomes on the counsellee's affective state, family members, current life circumstances and future; (b) explain that the test result can be refused if the individual has second thoughts about disclosure of such knowledge after the test is performed; and (c) provide a plan for post-test follow-up.	NG	As above

Autonomy/capacity

Grading	Evidence suggests that:	Type	Source
	Scores on mental status tests do not determine task-specific capacity.	NG	*ACCG, 1997b (from Post & Whitehouse, 1995)*
	Use of the terms competence and incompetence should be restricted to legal status, and legal judgements should reflect the mental condition of the person with dementia, not the needs or intolerance of others. Attending physicians routinely make non-legal (but probably valid) judgements of specific capacity, such as decisional capacity, based on common sense and observation.	NG	As above

Autonomy/capacity (continued)

Grading	Evidence suggests that:	Type	Source
	If an assessment of competency is required, the assessment should be undertaken by an individual or team which has special skill in making competency assessments. • The person's competence should be assessed only when there is a demonstrated need. • Assessment of an individual's competency should only be carried out in those domains in which an individual's competency is questioned.	NG	Alzheimer Society of Canada, 1992
	People with dementia should be allowed to exercise their remaining capacities for specific tasks and choices. Denying these choices challenges their independence and dignity.	NG	*ACCG, 1997a (from Post et al, 1997)*
	Autonomy can be extended prospectively through estate wills, living wills and durable powers of attorney for health care.	NG	*As above*
	Most commentators argue that standards of capacity assessment should vary with the likely harms or benefits that will follow from the decision.	NG	*As above*

Driving

Grading	Evidence suggests that:	Type	Source
***	Driving poses particular concern because of its public health impact. All patients and families should be informed that even mild dementia increases the risk of accidents.	EBG	APA, 1997
***	Advice about driving should be given to the family as well as the patient.	EBG	*As above*
**	Patients with mild impairments should be urged to stop driving or limit their driving to safer situations. Patients with moderate to severe impairments should be advised not to drive.	EBG	*As above*
	Driving cessation was associated with depressive symptoms among older persons.	CARS	*EBM, 1997e (from Marattoli et al, 1997)*
	Diagnosis of Alzheimer's disease is never itself sufficient reason for loss of driving privileges. The duty to prevent driving should not be applied prematurely or without individualised risk appraisal demonstrating impairment of driving ability.	NG	*ACCG, 1997b (from Post & Whitehouse, 1995)*

Quality of life

Driving (continued)

Grading	Evidence suggests that:	Type	Source
	The study considered the cost and effectiveness of a screening programme for older drivers (using the Mini-Mental State Examination; Folstein *et al*, 1975), beginning at the age of 65 years, compared with no screening programme. Six different strategies were considered: (a) no screening; (b) screening every five years; (c) screening every four years; (d) screening every three years; and (e) screening every two years; and (f) screening every year. The author considered only the incremental cost-effectiveness ratio for the annual screening programme, which was $2.9 million per life-year gained, since the other programmes were shown to have higher costs and lower benefits. (The NHS CRD database includes a commentary. Users of this information are strongly advised to look this up before altering their practice.)	EE	NEED; NHS CRD, 1998f (from Retchin *et al*, 1994)

Falls

Grading	Evidence suggests that:	Type	Source
***	Soft hip protector pads have been shown to dramatically reduce hip fractures in frail older people in residential care. Their effect and acceptability in the community needs further research.	SR	NHS CRD & Nuffield Institute of Health, 1996
***	There is some evidence to suggest that exercise, such as balance training, is effective in reducing the risk of falls in older people. Access to such interventions should be offered and ways of promoting uptake should be investigated. New programmes should be part of controlled evaluations.	SR	As above
***	High dose vitamin D supplementation with or without calcium appears to be effective in reducing fractures. Research is needed to identify the most cost-effective strategy.	SR	As above
***	Home visits and surveillance to assess and where appropriate, modify, environmental and personal risk factors can be effective in reducing falls. This can be carried out by nurses, health visitors, occupational therapists or trained volunteers.	SR	As above
**	Health care professionals should be aware that the risk of falls is not associated with the severity of the dementia but with the functional capability of the person, the risk being increased in the more capable group.	EBG	CHSR, 1998
**	Health care professionals should be aware that people with dementia who fall are more likely to fall again.	EBG	As above
**	Health care professionals should be aware of the factors contributing to the risk of falls which are medication, wandering and reversible confusion.	EBG	As above
**	Health care professionals should be aware that falls are increased in people with dementia.	EBG	As above

Falls (continued)

Grading	Evidence suggests that:	Type	Source
	The study examined the effect of different interventions, including different exercise regimes with resistance and/or endurance training, nutritional instruction, meditation and Tai Chi. The effect sizes in the study were not large, with effective treatments producing reductions in fall incidence of 10% and 17%. Tai Chi was notable in being more effective, but in small numbers. These effects, applied to the very large proportion of elderly people in today's society, would produce very significant benefits in falls and injuries avoided, would reduce disability and would allow considerable health care spending to be applied to more useful ends.	CARS	*Bandolier, 1995*
	A risk assessment score predicted which elderly patients would fall during a hospital stay.	CARS	*EBN*, 1998a (from Oliver *et al*, 1997)

Abuse

Grading	Evidence suggests that:	Type	Source
	The emphasis should be on preventing abuse by identifying and alleviating circumstances which are likely to lead to physical, psychosocial or financial abuse or neglect. <ul><li>Care-givers should be provided with education and training to enable them to give good care with little difficulty.</li><li>Care-givers should be provided with emotional supports, encouragement and care-giving assistance in order to reduce stress and burn-out.</li><li>When abuse has occurred, steps should be taken to prevent its recurrence.</li></ul>	NG	Alzheimer Society of Canada, 1992
	Care-givers should take action when they suspect abuse has occurred. <ul><li>Care-givers should be trained to identify cases of suspected abuse.</li><li>Paid care-givers should be familiar with the protocol on abuse in their facility or agency.</li></ul>	NG	As above
	Facilities and agencies should have a protocol on dealing with abuse. <ul><li>The protocol must protect the rights of the individual suspected of abuse, the rights of the abused person and the rights of the individual reporting the suspected abuse.</li><li>The protocol should describe a follow-up procedure to deal with the physical and emotional needs of the individual who has been abused.</li><li>The protocol should address the need for a written report of the incident and its contents.</li><li>The protocol should describe a procedure for following up with the alleged abuser, including the use of legal or disciplinary action.</li></ul>	NG	As above

Quality of life

Physical restraint

Grading	Evidence suggests that:	Type	Source
***	Physical restraints should be used only for patients who pose an imminent risk of physical harm to themselves or others and only until more definitive treatment is provided or when other measures have been exhausted.	EBG	APA, 1997
**	When restraints are used, the indications and alternatives should be carefully documented.	EBG	As above
**	The need for restraints can be decreased by environmental changes that decrease the risk of falls or wandering and by careful assessment and treatment of possible causes of agitation.	EBG	As above
	Every effort should be made to reduce the negative impact of the experience of being restrained and to preserve the person's dignity. • The application of a restraint should never be presented to the person as a punishment or a negative consequence of the person's behaviour. • If a restraint is the only method to ensure the safety of the individual or other people, the least restrictive method should be chosen. • The physical and emotional well-being of a person in a restrained condition should not be compromised.	NG	Alzheimer Society of Canada, 1992
	Every facility or agency should have a clearly stated protocol on the use of restraints. • The protocol should define the term restraint to include anything which limits an individual's voluntary movement. • The protocol should recognise that restraints are intrusive and an assault on an individual's dignity and freedom. • The protocol should clearly outline the circumstances under which restraints may be used and how their use will be monitored. • The protocol should be made available to the designated decision-maker at admission and should be discussed at that time.	NG	As above
	The emphasis should be on eliminating the need for restraints by preventing or managing the behaviour of concern. • A physical or chemical restraint should never be used as a substitute for a safe and well-designed environment and proper care and management of the person with Alzheimer's disease. • A restraint should never be used for the convenience of the care-giver. • Before using a restraint, care-givers should explore all alternative methods for dealing with the behaviour in question. • A restraint should not be considered a care option unless an assessment determines there is no other alternative to maintain the safety of the individual or others. • The behaviour for which the restraint is contemplated should have already occurred. • Before using a restraint, the relative danger of the behaviour versus the potential danger of applying a restraint should be considered and documented.	NG	As above
	Physical restraints result in unnecessary immobility and may be hazardous. Family care-givers should try to sustain the commitment to environmental and psychosocial methods of control.	NG	ACCG, 1997b (from Post & Whitehouse, 1995)

Carers and families

General

Grading	Evidence suggests that:	Type	Source
***	With the limited nature of the research evidence, it is not possible to recommend either wholesale investment in care-giver support programmes or withdrawal of the same.	SR	Thompson & Thompson, 1998
**	Health care professionals should be aware that referral of patients to respite and day care services may allow them to stay in their own home for longer.	EBG	CHSR, 1998
**	Health care professionals should be aware of the impact of caring for a person with dementia and the effect this has on the care-giver.	EBG	As above
**	Health care professionals should be aware that the impact of caring is dependent not on the severity of the cognitive impairment, but on the presentation of the dementia, e.g. factors such as behaviour and effect.	EBG	As above
	The study compared a care-giver support program for those caring for elderly relatives at home with two-level respite care, with conventional community nursing care. Because there was no statistically significant difference in individual item costs between the two groups, a 'conservative' incremental cost has been calculated based on the additional annual cost of the care-giver support program: the programme cost/care-giver/annum = £1240 (at 1991 prices).	EE	NEED; NHS CRD, 1998c (from Drummond *et al*, 1991)
	Outcome and cost duration was six months and the inclusion of treatment side-effects was not relevant. Incremental cost per quality-adjusted life year gained for the care-giver support program for those caring for elderly relatives at home, with two-level respite care was £12 365 (costs and benefits not discounted). (The NHS CRD database includes a commentary. Users of this information are strongly advised to look this up before altering their practice.)		
	Support for care-givers delayed nursing home placement of patients with Alzheimer's disease by almost a year.	CARS	CAT Bank; CEBM, 1997 (from Mittelman *et al*, 1996)
	Support for care-givers delayed time to nursing home placement in Alzheimer's disease.	CARS	*EBM*, 1997c (from Mittelman *et al*, 1996)

Information for parents and carers

Grading	Evidence suggests that:	Type	Source
**	Health care professionals should be aware that depressive illness is common in carers of people with dementia and is influenced by behavioural problems and higher care needs in the service user.	EBG	CHSR, 1998
	Physicians should inform the patient and their family about the probable diagnosis of Alzheimer's disease. This disclosure should ordinarily occur in a joint meeting and should allow time for questions and discussion. With disclosure comes responsibility to direct the patient and family to resources and to agree on a care plan. The utility of information from genetic testing has yet to be determined.	NG	ACCG, 1997b (from Post & Whitehouse, 1995)

Quality of life

Reducing carer distress/improving quality of life

Grading	Evidence suggests that:	Type	Source
***	Health care professionals should be aware that referral of patients to respite services offers satisfaction and relief to carers, although does not appear to alter the overall well-being of the carer.	EBG	CHSR, 1998
***	Health care professionals should be aware that referral of carers to groups for the provision of support and information about dementia is valued by the carer although unlikely to reduce the carer burden.	EBG	As above
***	Families and others often have great difficulty locating and arranging appropriate services for a person with dementia. This difficulty reflects the insufficient availability of some services, lack of funding for services, the complexity and fragmentation of services at the community level, the difficulty of obtaining accurate information about services, the difficulty of coordinating the services of multiple providers, and the characteristics, feelings and perceptions of some people with dementia and some family members that make them reluctant to use services. An effective system to link people with dementia to services has four components: public education, information and referral, case management and outreach.	HTA	HTA Database; NHS CRD, 1998a (from Office of Technology Assessment, 1990)
***	Care of dementia sufferers in homes decreases carer distress. The use of residential and nursing homes helps relieve carer distress. Part III homes and warden-supported homes are generally only used for those with milder forms of dementia. Care differs greatly from one establishment to another in terms of quality, staffing and programmes of care offered. The severity of dementia catered for also varies. There is a gradient of dependency from most severe in long-stay wards to least severe in residential and nursing homes. Many homes are reported to be inadequately staffed to meet the demands of people with dementia (e.g. behaviour problems, incontinence, wandering). This is particularly so in some residential homes where nursing staff may not be available. Studies suggest that many homes for people with dementia differ little from non-specialist homes for the elderly. Studies comparing specialist units (predominantly literature from the USA) suggest that in general carers prefer these units. There is no evidence to suggest that specialist units benefit people with dementia more than non-specialist units or wards, although non-sufferers may find the presence of large numbers of these patients distressing.	EBIP	Melzer et al, 1994
***	Use of long-term care in wards decreases carer distress. The quality of care varies enormously. Studies comparing long-term care on psychogeriatric wards to NHS nursing homes suggest that the two are comparable. There is no difference in their effect on cognitive function and carers report a similar decrease in level of distress.	EBIP	As above

Reducing carer distress/improving quality of life (continued)

Grading	Evidence suggests that:	Type	Source
**	Respite care relieves carer distress. Respite care covers a wide variety of programmes and settings. In assessing respite care, the programme offered must be clarified (respite care on demand, emergency or elective, length of time in care, frequency, duration of activities, specific therapies offered, etc). In combination with other community support services, respite care does help some carers manage the person at home for longer periods of time. Although it relieves carer distress, respite care is not suitable for every person with dementia as a proportion of people will become more confused as a result of being moved into a respite care facility. There is some suggestion that the degree of reduction of distress in carers is relatively modest. There is no indication of quantity, quality or content of care required within each severity category or patient/carer combination.	EBIP	Melzer et al, 1994
**	Health care professionals should be aware of the many factors contributing to the impact of caring and that male carers are less likely to complain spontaneously.	EBG	CHSR, 1998
**	Provision of information and counselling helps to reduce carer distress. Providing information and counselling aims to provide carers with an understanding of dementia, to reduce uncertainty, to develop effective coping techniques and hence reduce distress. There are many different models of providing information and counselling ranging from leaflets to intensive education and counselling in residential settings. The evidence for success of written guides is good, both in terms of use and practicality. One study of a comprehensive 10-day residential programme for both the patient and the carer showed a substantial decrease in hospital admissions and an increase in the length of time people remained in the community.	EBIP	Melzer et al, 1994
*	Health care professionals can improve satisfaction for carers by acknowledging and dealing with their distress and providing more information on dementia.	EBG	CHSR, 1998
*	Modest financial help is not associated with relieving distress in carers. Studies from the USA have shown that most care givers would prefer to receive appropriate free services than cash, perhaps because the amounts of financial assistance offered were too small to be of practical benefit.	EBIP	Melzer et al, 1994
*	Provision of substitution, enabling services and practical support helps to reduce carer distress and to assist with self-care of the dementia sufferer. These are services which assist in patient self-care and provide specific support to carers (e.g. 'meals on wheels', home help, health visiting, night-sitting, continence nurses, laundry service, etc). Substitution services are those replacing an activity the patient can no longer carry out (e.g. cooking, cleaning, shopping). It is clear that provision of these services	EBIP	As above

Quality of life

Reducing carer distress/improving quality of life (continued)

Grading	Evidence suggests that:	Type	Source
	does relieve carer burden and distress, and the greater the level of support, the greater the effect. There is little published work on the effectiveness of each service in isolation. The work which has been done suggests they are particularly useful in people with mild to moderate dementia who live alone.		
*	Day care has been shown to decrease carer distress. It is varied both in content and setting (e.g. hospital, day centre etc.). Content ranges from full programmes of activity and therapy to a sitting service. However, there is no evidence from the literature about what form day care should take, about levels of care in relation to outcomes, or about the amount of care required.	EBIP	Melzer *et al*, 1994
	Support for carers is a crucial part of the management of dementia. Carers should be encouraged to ventilate their feelings and, if possible, to share them with other carers and members of the primary care team as well as with family and friends. They may have high levels of psychiatric morbidity which may be reduced by improving support services or institutional care where appropriate. Carers also need to be aware of the natural history of the disease and that sudden deterioration requires a medical assessment to deter the underlying cause. Carers should be encouraged to join the Alzheimer's Disease Society which aims to give support to families by linking them through membership and self-help groups.	NG	Haines & Katona, 1992 (RCGP)
	All services should meet the needs of family care-givers as well as the needs of the person with Alzheimer's disease. • Communication with the family should be included in all aspects of all community- or facility-based services for people with sufferers. • Care-givers should be provided with information, counselling and support which is responsive to their needs. • Referrals to other agencies and support groups should be made as needed.	NG	Alzheimer Society of Canada, 1992
	All care-givers should have access to support and resources to relieve the work and stress which may result from caring for people with Alzheimer's disease. • A support or self-help group should be available to all care-givers. • Other psychosocial supports such as individual and group counselling should be available to all care-givers. • Care-givers should have access to information about resources and services which will help them provide care to the sufferer. • Administration in facilities and agencies should understand and support the special needs of staff providing care for sufferers.	NG	As above
	Courts should not remove the decision-making authority from families when no clear planning or documentation of advance directives have been completed.	NG	*ACCG, 1997b* (from Post & Whitehouse, 1995)

Clinical management

General

Grading	Evidence suggests that:	Type	Source
***	Another critical aspect of psychiatric management is educating the patient and family about the illness, its treatment and available sources of care and support (e.g. support groups, various types of respite care, nursing homes and other long-term care facilities, the Alzheimer's Association). It is also important to help patients and their families plan for financial and legal issues due to the patient's incapacity (e.g. power of attorney for medical and financial decisions, an up to date will, the cost of long-term care).	EBG	APA, 1997
	Health care professionals should exclude underlying causes of behavioural disorder e.g. an acute physical illness, environmental distress or physical discomfort.	EBG	CHSR, 1998
	The mainstays of management in established dementia are: • to identify specific problems (e.g. incontinence, progression – remember there may be other concurrent causes) and strategies to improve them; • to preserve existing functioning; and • to provide adequate overall care for the patient and his or her network of informal support.	NG	Haines & Katona, 1992 (RCGP)

Coexisting mental health problems

Depression

Grading	Evidence suggests that:	Type	Source
**	Depressed mood may respond to improvements in the living situation or stimulation-oriented treatments.	EBG	APA, 1997
**	Although research data are limited, clinical experience suggests that electroconvulsive therapy (ECT) is effective in the treatment of patients with depression who do not respond to other agents.	EBG	As above
*	ECT may be effective for dementia patients who are suffering from depression. Twice- rather than thrice-weekly and unilateral rather than bilateral treatments may decrease the risk of delirium or memory loss associated with this modality.	EBG	As above

Clinical management

Psychosis and agitation

Grading	Evidence suggests that:	Type	Source
***	Psychosis and agitation are common in patients with dementia, often coexist, and may respond to similar therapies. In approaching any of these symptoms, it is critical to consider the safety of the patient and those around him or her.	EBG	APA, 1997
***	After ensuring safety, the next step is a careful evaluation for a general medical, psychiatric or psychosocial problem that may underlie the disturbance. If attention to these issues does not resolve the problem and the symptoms do not cause undue distress to the patient or others, they are best treated with reassurance and distraction.	EBG	As above

Sleep problems

Grading	Evidence suggests that:	Type	Source
***	Pharmacological interventions should be considered only when other interventions, including careful attention to sleep hygiene, have failed.	EBG	APA, 1997
**	If a patient has a sleep disturbance and requires medication for another condition, an agent with sedating properties, given at bedtime, should be selected if possible.	EBG	As above
**	Diphenhydramine is generally not recommended because of its anticholinergic properties.	EBG	As above
**	If the sleep disturbance does not coexist with other problems, potentially effective agents include zolpidem and trazodone, but there are few data on the efficacy of specific agents for patients with dementia.	EBG	As above
**	Benzodiazepine and chloral hydrate are usually not recommended for other than for brief use because of the risk of daytime sedation, tolerance, rebound insomnia, worsening cognition, disinhibition and delirium.	EBG	As above
**	Triazolam in particular is not recommended because of its association with amnesia.	EBG	As above
	Sleep disturbances are common in patients with dementia.	EBG	As above

Physical screening/care

General			
Grading	Evidence suggests that:	Type	Source
***	It is particularly critical to identify and treat general medical conditions that may be responsible for or contribute to the dementia or associated behavioural symptoms.	EBG	APA, 1997
**	Health care professionals should be aware of the existence of reversible causes of dementia.	EBG	CHSR, 1998
**	GPs should ensure that the following routine tests are performed: haematology (including erythrocyte sedimentation rate), biochemistry, bone chemistry, thyroid function and simple urinalysis.	EBG	As above
**	Health care professionals should be aware that people with dementia experience physical morbidity to the same degree as the general population but are likely to under-report their symptoms.	EBG	As above
	In the case of multi-infarct dementia, control of risk factors (hypertension, smoking, obesity, diabetes) may improve cognitive function as well as reducing the risk of re-infarction. It is equally important to reduce these risk factors in patients liable to develop multi-infarct dementia.	NG	Haines & Katona, 1992 (RCGP)

Follow-up, monitoring, assessment

General			
Grading	Evidence suggests that:	Type	Source
***	More frequent visits (e.g. once or twice a week) may be required for patients with complex or potentially dangerous symptoms or during the administration of specific therapies.	EBG	APA, 1997
**	In order to offer prompt treatment, assure safety and provide timely advice to the patient and family, it is generally necessary to see patients in routine follow-up every four to six months.	EBG	As above
	Frequency of follow-up might vary from four to six months in the case of a patient whose condition is stable and who has a well-established support network, to every two weeks or so in the case of an isolated patient, or one with inadequate support.	NG	Haines & Katona, 1992 (RCGP)
	Frequency of monitoring depends on the severity of the patient's condition, the presence or absence of carers (both professional and informal) and whether or not the patient attends a day centre or other facility.	NG	As above
	Surveillance of the elderly population is greatly facilitated by the use of an elderly 'at risk' register, which can be compiled from the general practice age/gender register.	NG	As above

Clinical management

General (continued)			
Grading	*Evidence suggests that:*	*Type*	*Source*
	Monitoring may include repeat testing of cognitive function using the Abbreviated Mental Test Score (Hodkinson, 1972), or another suitable instrument, to determine whether deterioration is occurring. Routine questioning and examinations are indicated to detect intercurrent problems, particularly urinary and faecal incontinence, dehydration, constipation, evidence of inadequate nutrition, anaemia and cardiac failure. Regular functional assessment is valuable in determining whether the patient and carer need extra support. This includes asking whether patients need assistance with personal care routines such as washing and bathing, feeding, cutting of nails, toileting and dressing, as well as home care tasks, such as cooking, cleaning, shopping, paying bills and collecting pensions. Knowledge of the patient's mobility is also vital, including whether the patient can get in and out of a chair, walk on the flat or upstairs, whether the patient wanders or exhibits any other dangerous behaviour.	NG	Haines & Katona, 1992 (RCGP)
	Follow-up also provides an opportunity to assess the carer's response to changing circumstances. Evidence of depression or other psychiatric morbidity in the carer may be an indication for greater professional support.	NG	As above
	The most crucial aspect of follow-up is determining who will take primary responsibility. The psychogeriatric department, the GP, the community psychiatric nurse, the nurse adviser to the elderly or district nurse are all potential candidates in individual cases.	NG	As above

Prognosis

General			
Grading	*Evidence suggests that:*	*Type*	*Source*
	Dementia severity, wandering and falling and behavioural problems were associated with shorter survival in Alzheimer's disease.	CARS	*ACP Journal Club*, 1991a (from Walsh *et al*, 1990)
	Algorithms provided useful information about the course of Alzheimer's disease.	CARS	*ACP Journal Club*, 1997a (from Stern *et al*, 1997

Death

General			
Grading	Evidence suggests that:	Type	Source
	The physician should initiate discussion about use of aggressive life-prolonging measures.	NG	ACCG, 1997b (from Post & Whitehouse, 1995
	A 'good' death requires that the patient's values be integrated into the process of dying.	NG	As above
	The philosophy of hospice is highly appropriate for the care of people with advanced dementia.	NG	As above
	People with Alzheimer's disease have a terminal illness, although death will usually result from pneumonia and other causes that the illness precipitates.	NG	As above

Psychosocial interventions

General			
Grading	Evidence suggests that:	Type	Source
*	Non-drug interventions should always be considered along with drug options before treatment is started.	EBG	SIGN, 1998
	Non-drug management (apart from specific psychological approaches such as reminiscence therapy and reality orientation, which may be available through the psychogeriatric services) consists mainly of appropriate service provision.	NG	Haines & Katona, 1992 (RCGP)

Programmes and activities			
Grading	Evidence suggests that:	Type	Source
	Programmes for persons with Alzheimer's disease should include the routines of daily living as well as special activities. • Programmes should include the performance of basic self-care, opportunities for social interaction and events traditionally identified as 'activities'. • Individuals should have the opportunity to pursue familiar activities which reflect their habitual lifestyle and interests.	NG	Alzheimer Society of Canada, 1992

Psychosocial interventions

Programmes and activities (continued)

Grading	Evidence suggests that:	Type	Source
	Programmes serving people with Alzheimer's disease should promote well-being and enjoyment, respond to the individual's physical, emotional, spiritual and sensory needs and encourage as much autonomy as possible. • Programmes should provide for quiet, private times as well as group interactions. • All activities and interpersonal encounters should reflect respect for the person's status as an adult and an individual. • Activities should be satisfying and promote a sense of trust and mastery. • The programme should offer the individual the opportunity to use abilities and to handle familiar objects.	NG	Alzheimer Society of Canada, 1992
	Activities that creatively draw on remaining abilities (e.g. art and music) can influence behaviour positively.	NG	ACCG, 1997b (from Post & Whitehouse, 1995
	Programmes and activities should be flexible and change in response to the changing needs of the person with Alzheimer's disease. • The individual's response to programmes and activities should be documented and reviewed regularly with members of the care team. • The response to programmes and activities should be included as part of the care plan review.	NG	Alzheimer Society of Canada, 1992

Psychological therapies

General

Grading	Evidence suggests that:	Type	Source
***	No firm conclusions on the effectiveness of reminiscence therapy for dementia can be reached, because only one randomised controlled trial has been used. Other literature suggests that for potential benefits of reminiscence therapy to be sustained, it should be part of an ongoing programme, or features of it should become part of daily activities.	SR	Spector & Orrell, 1998a
***	There is some evidence that reality orientation has benefits on both cognition and behaviour for dementia sufferers. Further research could examine which features of reality orientation are particularly effective. It is unclear how far the benefits of reality orientation extend after the end of treatment, but some evidence suggests that a continued programme may be needed to sustain potential benefits.	SR	Spector & Orrell, 1998b
***	Overall, elderly subjects treated with any form of therapy (reality orientation, cognitive training, physical exercise, socialisation, reminiscence and interactive contact or touch) tended to improve. Of the 79 effect sizes calculated, 85% were positive. The large differences in the effect sizes across types of treatments and types of outcome measures inferred that some treatments work better than others and that some patient outcomes are more easily influenced than others. (The NHS CRD database includes a commentary. Users of this information are strongly recommended to look this up before altering their practice).	NG	DARE; NHS CRD, 1998g (from Burckhardt, 1987)

Grading	Evidence suggests that:	Type	Source

General (continued)

Grading	Evidence suggests that:	Type	Source
**	A range of therapies (reality orientation, cognitive stimulation and validation therapy) are used to keep the person mentally alert although none have shown more than marginal effect. Studies of each specific therapy have been largely evaluated on institutionalised patients. Reality orientation has had some success in people with dementia, improving orientation for time, place and person but it has little effect on behavioural problems. There is also evidence suggesting that speech and language therapy is beneficial to those with dementia (and may form part of the initial assessment).	EBIP	Melzer *et al*, 1994
*	Among the emotion-oriented treatments, supportive psychotherapy is used by some practitioners to address issues of loss in the early stages of dementia, reminiscence therapy has some modest research support for improvement of mood and behaviour while validation therapy and sensory integration have less research support. None of these modalities has been subjected to rigorous testing.	EBG	APA, 1997
*	Cognition-oriented treatments focused on specific cognitive deficits, such as reality orientation, cognitive retraining and skills training, are unlikely to be beneficial, and have been associated with frustration in some patients.	EBG	As above

Behaviour-oriented interventions

General

Grading	Evidence suggests that:	Type	Source
**	Behaviour-oriented treatments identify the antecedents and consequences of problem behaviours and institute changes in the environment that minimise precipitants and/or consequences. These approaches have not been subjected to randomised clinical trials but are supported by single-case studies and are in widespread clinical use.	EBG	APA, 1997

Stimulation-oriented interventions

General

Grading	Evidence suggests that:	Type	Source
**	Stimulation-oriented treatments, such as recreational activity, art therapy and pet therapy, along with other formal and informal means of maximising pleasurable activities for patients, have modest support from clinical trials for improving function and mood, and common sense supports their use as part of the humane care of patients with dementia.	EBG	APA, 1997

Psychosocial interventions

45

Multi-disciplinary team interventions

General			
Grading	*Evidence suggests that:*	*Type*	*Source*
***	The objective of the review was to determine the effectiveness, if any, of multi-disciplinary team interventions in the coordinated care of patients with delirium superimposed on an underlying chronic cognitive impairment compared with the usual care of older patients with cognitive impairments. Insufficient data are available for the development of evidence-based guidelines on diagnosis, or management.	SR	Britton & Russell, 1998

Medication

General			
Grading	*Evidence suggests that:*	*Type*	*Source*
***	The elderly and patients with dementia are more sensitive to certain medication side-effects, including anticholinergic effects, orthostasis, central nervous system sedation and parkinsonism.	EBG	APA, 1997
***	Psychoactive medications are effective in the management of some symptoms associated with dementia, but they must be used with caution.	EBG	As above
***	Medications should be used with considerable care, particularly when more than one agent is being used.	EBG	As above
***	There is no effective drug marketed for the prevention or relief of the more common types of dementia. However, there is much active research in this field at present. Drugs are successfully used to control behavioural problems, sleeplessness and associated depression.	EBIP	Melzer et al, 1994
**	Elderly individuals have decreased renal clearance and slowed hepatic metabolism of many medications, so lower starting doses, smaller increases in dose and longer intervals between increments must be used.	EBG	APA, 1997
**	General medical conditions and other medications may further alter the binding, metabolism and excretion of many medications.	EBG	As above
	Where underlying causes are identified they should be managed before prescribing for a behavioural disorder.	EBG	CHSR, 1998
	Behaviour-controlling drugs should be used cautiously and only for specified purposes, with as few drugs as possible at low dosages with increases in doses monitored for side-effects. Used carefully for defined goals (such as keeping the patient at home), drugs can be highly beneficial.	NG	ACCG, 1997b (from Post & Whitehouse, 1995

Antidepressants

Grading	Evidence suggests that:	Type	Source
***	Antidepressants can have many side-effects, including sedation, worsening cognition, delirium, an increase in the risk of falls and worsening of sleep-disordered breathing.	EBG	APA, 1997
***	Agents with significant anticholinergic effects (e.g. amitriptyline and imipramine) should be avoided.	EBG	As above
***	The choice among agents is based on the side-effect profile and the characteristics of a given patient.	EBG	As above
**	Because of the elevated risk of dietary indiscretion in patients with dementia and the substantial risk of postural hypotension, monoamine oxidase inhibitors are probably appropriate only for patients who have not responded to other treatments.	EBG	As above
**	Consider a trial of antidepressant medication at a therapeutic dose evaluated against explicit criteria such as activities of daily living, level of functioning, behavioural disturbance and biological features of recent onset.	EBG	CHRS, 1998
**	Consider antidepressant medication for marked and persistent depression.	EBG	SIGN, 1998
**	Selective serotonin reuptake inhibitors (SSRIs) are probably the first-line treatment, although one of the tricyclic antidepressants or newer agents, such as bupropion or venlafaxine, may be more appropriate for some patients.	EBG	APA, 1997
**	Although formal evaluation of the efficacy of antidepressants for patients with dementia is limited, there is considerable clinical evidence supporting their use.	EBG	As above
**	Lithium and beta-blockers are not generally recommended. The few data supporting their use concern populations not affected by dementia, and the potential side-effects are serious.	EBG	As above
*	Patients with severe or persistent depressed mood with or without a full complement of neurovegetative signs should be treated with antidepressant medications.	EBG	As above
*	The anticonvulsant agents carbamazepine and valproate, the sedating antidepressant trazodone, the atypical anxiolytic busprone and possibly SSRIs are less well-studied but may be appropriate for patients without psychosis affected by behavioural disorders, especially those with mild symptoms or sensitivity to antipsychotic medications. There is preliminary evidence to support their efficacy in the treatment of agitation.	EBG	As above
	Moclobemide was an effective antidepressant in elderly patients with cognitive decline and depression.	CARS	*EBM*, 1996 (from Roth *et al*, 1996)

Medication

Anxiolytics

Grading	Evidence suggests that:	Type	Source
**	Benzodiazepines are most useful for treating patients with prominent anxiety, or for giving on an as-needed basis to patients who have infrequent episodes of agitation or to individuals who need to be sedated for a procedure such as a tooth extraction.	EBG	APA, 1997
**	A structured education programme for staff may decrease the use of antidepressant medications in nursing homes.	EBG	As above
**	Benzodiazepines appear to perform better than placebo but not as well as antipsychotics in treating behavioural symptoms, although the data are of limited quality.	EBG	As above
*	It may be preferable to use lorazepam and oxazepam, which have no active metabolites and are not metabolised in the liver.	EBG	As above
*	Consider short-term anxiolytic or hypnotic treatment for severe and persistent symptoms.	EBG	SIGN, 1998
	Triazolam caused sedation and impairment of psychomotor performance in elderly people.	CARS	*ACP Journal Club*, 1991d (from Greenblatt *et al*, 1991)

Antipsychotics

Grading	Evidence suggests that:	Type	Source
***	Antipsychotics have a number of potentially severe side-effects, including sedation and worsening of cognition, and thus must be used at the lowest effective dose. Extremely low starting doses are recommended for this population.	EBG	APA, 1997
***	High-potency agents are more likely to cause akathisia and Parkinsonian symptoms. Low-potency agents are more likely to cause sedation, confusion, delirium, postural hypotension and peripheral anticholinergic effects.	EBG	As above
***	Clozapine is much less likely to be associated with extrapyramidal reactions, but it is associated with sedation, postural hypotension and an elevated seizure risk and carries a risk of agranulocytosis. It therefore requires regular monitoring of blood counts.	EBG	As above
***	Antipsychotics are the only documented pharmacological treatment for psychosis in dementia.	EBG	As above
***	The decision of which antipsychotic to use is based on the relationship between the side-effect profile and the characteristics of a given patient.	EBG	As above
***	When used appropriately, antipsychotics can relieve symptoms and reduce distress for patients and can increase safety for patients, other residents and staff.	EBG	As above

Antipsychotics *(continued)*

Grading	Evidence suggests that:	Type	Source
***	Over-use of antipsychotic medication can lead to worsening of the dementia, over-sedation, falls and tardive dyskinesia. Thus, federal regulations and good clinical practice require careful consideration and documentation of the indications and available alternatives, both initially and at other times.	EBG	APA, 1997
***	A dose decrease or discontinuation should be considered periodically for all patients who receive antipsychotic medications.	EBG	As above
***	Antipsychotics have been shown to provide modest improvement in behavioural symptoms in general.	EBG	As above
**	Treatment should normally be short-term and should be reviewed regularly.	EBG	SIGN, 1998
**	Some research evidence, along with considerable anecdotal evidence, suggests that any improvement is greater for psychosis than for other symptoms.	EBG	APA, 1997
**	There is no evidence of a difference in efficacy between antipsychotic agents.	EBG	As above
**	The efficacy of these agents beyond eight weeks has limited research support, but there is considerable clinical experience with this practice.	EBG	As above
**	Antipsychotics are best documented for agitation.	EBG	As above
**	Neuroleptics should normally be avoided where there is a possibility of Lewy Body type dementia.	EBG	SIGN, 1998
**	Dose should be reduced as soon as possible and treatment stopped if no longer essential.	EBG	As above
**	Patients known to have dementia with Lewy Bodies should not be treated with neuroleptics.	EBG	CHSR, 1998
**	Health care professionals should be aware of the importance of avoiding the use of neuroleptic agents in people known to have dementia with Lewy Bodies.	EBG	As above
**	Low doses should be prescribed initially, with slow and cautious increase as necessary: 'start low, go slow'.	EBG	SIGN, 1998
*	Risperidone appears to share the risks associated with high-potency agents, although it may be somewhat less likely to cause extrapyramidal reactions.	EBG	APA, 1997
*	Neuroleptics should only be considered for patients with serious problems, in particular psychotic symptoms, or in the presence of serious distress or danger from behaviour disturbance.	EBG	SIGN, 1998
	In crisis situations the short-term use of neuroleptics may be appropriate.	EBG	CHSR, 1998

Medication

Antipsychotics (continued)

Grading	Evidence suggests that:	Type	Source
	Neuroleptics have been widely used but evidence for their efficacy is limited.	EBG	SIGN, 1998
	Side-effect profiles differ.	EBG	SIGN, 1998
	All conventional antipsychotic agents are also associated with more serious complications, including tardive dyskinesia (for which the elderly, women, and individuals with dementia are at increased risk) and neuroleptic malignant syndrome.	EBG	APA, 1997
	There is no clear evidence for the superiority of one neuroleptic drug over any other.	EBG	SIGN, 1998
	Drug treatment should be aimed mainly at controlling behaviour and treating causes of acute deterioration. Major tranquillisers may be useful to reduce disinhibition, aggression or wandering, but may cause considerable sedation, extrapyramidal movement disorder and increased confusion. In general, all drugs should be titrated against response to achieve the lowest effective dose and reviewed regularly. Polypharmacy is particularly likely to lead to adverse effects in patients with dementia, and compliance is often a problem.	NG	Haines & Katona, 1992 (RCGP)

Donepezil and tacrine

Grading	Evidence suggests that:	Type	Source
***	Tacrine has been shown to lead to modest improvements in cognition in a substantial minority of patients, but up to 30% of patients cannot tolerate the medication because of nausea and vomiting or substantial (but reversible) elevations in liver enzyme levels.	EBG	APA, 1997
***	In the light of limited current knowledge, general practitioners should not initiate treatment with donepezil.	EBG	CHSR, 1997
***	There is no convincing evidence that tacrine is a useful treatment for the symptoms of Alzheimer's disease. However, as so few trials presented data in a format suitable for pooling, the results of this review may be modified when further data from all relevant trials are included.	SR	Quizilbash *et al*, 1998a
***	In the light of limited current knowledge, general practitioners should not continue hospital-initiated treatment with donepezil.	EBG	CHSR, 1998
***	In the light of current knowledge, tacrine should not be used by general practitioners for the treatment of dementia.	EBG	CHSR, 1998
***	Evidence to support the use of donepezil in the treatment of mild to moderate senile dementia of the Alzheimer type, is borderline. • Evidence is limited in quantity and by restriction to a select population. • There is evidence of temporary benefit but at considerable cost. • Treatment should be targeted carefully. Any protocol for its use should include clear criteria and a review within two to three months. • Further research is needed.	SR	Stein, 1997 (Wessex Institute)

Donepezil and tacrine (continued)

Grading	Evidence suggests that:	Type	Source
***	Two cholinersterase inhibitors are available for Alzheimer's disease: tacrine and donepezil. Either may be offered to patients with mild to moderate Alzheimer's disease after a thorough discussion of its potential risks and benefits.	EBG	APA, 1997
*	Because donepezil does not share tacrine's risk for liver toxicity, and thus does not require frequent monitoring, it may prove preferable as a first-line treatment. (However, accumulated data from additional clinical trials and clinical practice will be necessary in order to establish a more complete picture of its efficacy and side-effect profile).	EBG	As above
	Donepezil improved cognitive and global function in mild to moderate Alzheimer's disease.	CARS	*EBMH*, 1998b (from Rogers *et al*, 1998)
	High-dose tacrine improved symptoms in patients with Alzheimer's disease.	CARS	*ACP Journal Club*, 1994 (from Knapp *et al*, 1994)
	Current therapies slow but do not prevent the progression of Alzheimer's disease. This study indicates that, over the short-term, donepezil 5 mg/day is a safe and effective treatment for slowing the decline of patients with mild to moderate Alzheimer's disease. Long term benefit, especially in patients with comorbid conditions, and cost effectiveness need to be determined before recommending the routine use of donepezil in patients with Alzheimer's disease.	CARS	*Journal of Evidence-Based Practice POEM*, 1998 (from Rogers *et al*, 1998)
	Donepezil is an expensive new drug for the treatment of dementia, costing about £1000 per patient per year. It is difficult to find a definition of a clinically useful outcome, the number of patients who benefited and whether that benefit was sustained in those patients. There was a small average decline in the Alzheimer Disease Assessment Score (ADAS-Cog) in those receiving placebo (of 0.7 on a 70-point scale, with a range of change from a fall of seven points to an increase of 14.5 points), and a small average increase in those on 5 mg donepezil (2.5 on a 70-point scale, with a range of change from a fall of eight points to an increase of seven points). The difference was statistically significant.	CARS	*Bandolier*, 1997
	The Standing Medical Advisory Committee recommends that treatment with donepezil should be initiated and supervised only by a specialist experienced in the management of dementia. Benefit should be assessed at 12 weeks. Treatment should continue only for those patients with evidence of benefit.	NG	Standing Medical Advisory Committee (DOH), 1998

Medication

51

Ergot mesylates

Grading	Evidence suggests that:	Type	Source
***	Co-dergocrine mesylate is not sufficiently effective to be routinely recommended as a treatment for dementia.	EBG	CHSR, 1997
***	Ergot mesylates has no significant side-effects.	EBG	APA, 1997
***	Co-dergocrine mesylate shows significant treatment effects when assessed by either global gradings or comprehensive grading scales. The small number of trials available for analysis, however, limited the ability of subgroup analyses to identify statistically significant moderating effects. Other methodological problems mean that there is still uncertainty regarding co-dergocrine mesylate's efficacy in dementia.	SR	Olin *et al*, 1998
*	The mixture of ergot mesylates cannot be recommended for the treatment of cognitive symptoms but may be offered to patients with vascular dementia and may be appropriately continued for patients who experience a benefit.	EBG	APA, 1997
*	Ergot mesylates has been assessed in a large number of studies with inconsistent findings, but there is a suggestion that it may have more benefit for patients with vascular dementia than those with degenerative dementias.	EBG	As above
	Co-dergocrine mesylate is effective for dementia. It is more effective than placebo in patients with vascular dementia, in in-patients compared with out-patients, and in higher compared with lower dosages. It has modest effects in patients with Alzheimer's disease. The conditions for obtaining benefits from co-dergocrine mesylate are inadequately defined.	CARS	*ACP Journal Club*, 1995 (from Schneider & Olin, 1994)

Selegiline and vitamin E

Grading	Evidence suggests that:	Type	Source
***	Although the evidence for a beneficial effect of selegiline on patients with Alzheimer's disease is promising, there is not yet enough evidence to recommend its routine use in practice.	SR	Birks & Flicker, 1998
***	The role of selegiline in the treatment of Alzheimer's disease has still to be established by large well-controlled, long-term clinical trials. The trials reviewed in this study infer that selegiline may be a useful agent in managing behavioural and cognitive symptomatology. In the absence of a standard treatment and given that the treatment of Alzheimer's disease is symptomatic, selegiline should be considered among other alternative treatments. (The NHS CRD database includes a commentary. Users of this information are strongly advised to look this up before altering their practice).	SR	DARE; NHS CRD, 1998h (from Tolbert & Fuller, 1996
***	Vitamin E may be considered for patients with moderate Alzheimer's disease to prevent further decline.	EBG	APA, 1997
***	Because there is no evidence of an additive effect of vitamin E and selegiline, there is no empirical basis for using the two agents in combination.	EBG	As above

Selegiline and vitamin E (continued)

Grading	Evidence suggests that:	Type	Source
***	A single large well-constructed trial of vitamin E showed a significant delay in poor outcome over a two-year period and the agent appears to be very safe.	EBG	APA, 1997
***	A single large well-conducted trial of selegiline showed a significant delay in poor outcome over a two-year period.	EBG	As above
**	Vitamin E might be considered alone or in combination with an anticholinergic agent in the treatment of Alzheimer's disease.	EBG	As above
**	Selegiline may be considered for patients with moderate Alzheimer's disease to prevent further decline.	EBG	As above
**	Selegiline is associated with orthostatic hypotension and a risk for medication interactions, so vitamin E, which appeared equally efficacious in a direct comparison, may be preferable.	EBG	As above
*	As well as for patients with moderate Alzheimer's disease, vitamin E might also be beneficial earlier or later in the course of the disease.	EBG	As above
*	Because limited evidence suggests that selegiline may offer short-term improvement in dementia, it may be appropriate as an alternative to cholinersterase inhibitors in patients who are ineligible for, intolerant of, or unresponsive to these agents.	EBG	As above
*	Selegiline may possibly be beneficial earlier (before the patient has moderate disease) or later in the course of the disease.	EBG	As above
	Selegiline and α-tocopherol (vitamin E) slowed the progression of Alzheimer's disease.	CARS	*EBM, 1997d* (from Sano et al, 1997)
	This study examined whether selegiline, α-tocopherol or a combination of both drugs slowed the progression of Alzheimer's disease of moderate severity. Results suggested that selegiline and vitamin E can improve behavioural symptoms etc. The POEM commentator argues that while improvements are statistically significant, they are not clinically significant and that outcome measures used may not be appropriate. The commentator indicates the following recommendations for practice: "I would consider trying vitamin E in patients with moderately severe AD since it can be obtained over-the-counter, and is relatively non-toxic and inexpensive".	CARS	*Journal of Evidence-Based Practice POEM, 1997c* (from Sano et al, 1997)

Medication

Ginkgo biloba

Grading	Evidence suggests that:	Type	Source
	Seven patients have to be treated with 120 mg of Ginkgo extract daily for one year for one of them to have an improved Alzheimer Disease Assessment Score (ADAS-Cog) of four points which they would not have had with placebo. For a two-point improvement, about four patients have to be treated for one year. For a patient's family member to notice an improvement in their daily living and social behaviour about seven patients have to be treated for one year.	CARS	*Bandolier, 1998*
	Ginkgo biloba (EGb 761) appears to have a modest stabilising effect on the general functional decline of otherwise healthy patients with dementia. EGb appeared to be as safe as placebo, although the small number of patients and the short time period limits the ability to detect uncommon events. The changes reported are of a similar magnitude to those seen with tacrine and donepezil, two currently available medications that, locally, cost three times more than Gingko extracts. Whether EGb is safer or more effective than these medications is not clear. Recommendations to patients should be made with caution, since Gingko biloba does not face the regulatory scrutiny of prescription medications. Nonetheless, it appears that EGb may have some beneficial effects in demented individuals.	CARS	*Journal of Evidence-Based Practice* POEM, *1997b* (from Le Bars *et al*, 1997)
	Gingko biloba safely and modestly improved dementia.	CARS	*EBM*, *1998b* (from Le Bars *et al*, 1997)

Hormones

Grading	Evidence suggests that:	Type	Source
*	Medroxyprogesterone and related hormones may have a role in the treatment of disinhibited sexual behaviour in male patients with dementia.	EBG	APA, 1997
	Post-menopausal oestrogen reduced the risk for and delayed the onset of Alzheimer's disease.	CARS	*EBM*, *1997b* (from Tang *et al*, 1996)

Psychostimulants

Grading	Evidence suggests that:	Type	Source
*	Treatments for apathy are not well-documented but psychostimulants, bupropion, bromocriptine and amantadine may be helpful.	EBG	APA, 1997
*	Psychostimulants are also sometimes useful in the treatment of depression in patients with significant general medical illness.	EBG	As above

Other

Grading	Evidence suggests that:	Type	Source
***	The data at present offer limited support for improvement in a sense of well-being following DHEA treatment. The data offer no support at present for improvement in memory or other aspects of cognitive function following DHEA treatment.	SR	Huppert *et al*, 1998
***	There is some evidence that cytidinediphosphocholine (CDP-choline) has a positive effect on memory and behaviour in at least the short term. The evidence of benefit from global impression is stronger, but is still limited by the duration of the studies. There is evidence that the effect of treatment is more homogeneous for patients with cognitive impairment secondary to cerebrovascular disorder.	SR	Fioravanti & Yanagi, 1998
***	At this stage the evidence available from the published literature does not support the use of piracetam in the treatment of people with dementia or cognitive impairment because effects were found only on global impression of change but not on any of the more specific measures.	SR	Flicker & Grimley-Evans, 1998
***	There is no convincing evidence that nimodipine is a useful treatment for the symptoms of dementia, either unclassified or according to the major subtypes – Alzheimer's disease, vascular or mixed Alzheimer's and vascular dementia. Nimodipine cannot be currently recommended for patients with dementia.	SR	Qizilbash *et al*, 1998b
***	Evidence from randomised trials does not support the use of lecithin in the treatment of patients with dementia or cognitive impairment. A moderate effect cannot be ruled out, but results from the small trials to date do not indicate priority for a large randomised trial.	SR	Higgins & Flicker, 1998
***	Vasodilators should not be prescribed as a treatment for dementia.	EBG	CHSR, 1998
**	Health care professionals should be aware that a reduction in risk of further vascular events for people who have early dementia known to be related to cerebral ischaemia may be achieved by treating with aspirin 75 mg. The size of any effect on cognitive impairment is unclear.	EBG	As above
*	Routine use of anticholinergic medication to prevent extrapyramidal side-effects is not appropriate.	EBG	SIGN, 1998
*	Risk of side-effects must be balanced against any perceived benefit.	EBG	As above
*	A variety of other agents have been suggested as possibly helpful in the treatment of cognitive symptoms, some of the most promising of which are under active study in clinical trials. Because these agents remain experimental, they are best taken in the context of a clinical trial. Such trials may be an appropriate option for some patients, since they offer the chance of clinical benefit while contributing to progress in treating dementia.	EBG	APA, 1997

Medication

Other (continued)

Grading	Evidence suggests that:	Type	Source
	Acetyl-L-carnitine treatment was associated with a deceleration of the decline in behavioural and cognitive abilities in patients with Alzheimer's disease. Acetyl-L-carnitine warrants further larger trials of longer duration.	CARS	*ACP Journal Club*, 1992 (from Spagnoli *et al*, 1991)
	Non-steroidal anti-inflammatory drugs, but not aspirin or acetaminophen, reduced the risk for Alzheimer's disease.	CARS	*ACP Journal Club*, 1997b (from Stewart *et al*, 1997)
	Intramuscular desferrioxamine slowed the decline in living skills in Alzheimer's disease.	CARS	*ACP Journal Club*, 1991b (from McClachlan *et al*, 1991)

Organisation of care

Referral

Grading	Evidence suggests that:	Type	Source
	All patients with dementia may be referred to a psychogeriatrician or geriatrician at least for initial assessment, after which they may be referred back to the care of the GP. This could create a considerable burden on services, however, systematic screening is being undertaken as part of the annual check for patients aged 75 years and over. Some GPs may prefer to keep the initial management and assessment in their own hands. Social factors are also a major consideration in the decision whether or not to refer a patients.	NG	Haines & Katona, 1992 (RCGP)
	If there is a specific indication for specialised continuing assessment, or therapeutic intervention focused on patients with dementia themselves and/or their carers, they should be followed up by a multi-disciplinary psychogeriatric team where available.	NG	As above
	A demand for respite care is another important indication for referral because of the need to prevent breakdown in the carer's ability to cope with the patient which may in turn lead to long-term institutionalisation. Admissions for respite care need to be planned well in advance. Therefore early referral is recommended if respite care is likely to be needed.	NG	As above
	A sudden onset of confusion or sudden deterioration in the state of a person with dememtia requires medical assessment to exclude causes such as urinary infection, faecal impaction, chest infection and side-effects of drugs. Failure to find a cause for the deterioration, or failure of the patient to respond to treatment of the apparent cause, is an indication for referral.	NG	As above

Referral (continued)

Grading	Evidence suggests that:	Type	Source
	Easy and early referral should be encouraged by the service, and telephone referral – giving sufficient detail to the secretary – should be acceptable. Appropriate letter referral from the GP is also to be encouraged. Locally publicised information for GPs on optimum referral information and on how to facilitate referral is helpful. Some services use answerphones and helplines to facilitate more open contact but, particularly with patients in the community, it is always important that the GP be involved at the earliest stage.	NG	RCPsych, 1995
	The service should establish the medically perceived reasonable timescale in which assessment is required and offer to meet this, including a very urgent response (same-day) when necessary. With most cases a more routine response will be agreed. An accepted timescale, within which all referrals will usually be seen, is useful. This may be one week, or 10 days for instance, but should not be more than two to three weeks. With particular cases, perhaps for some out-patients, a longer timescale may be agreed.	NG	As above
	Normally referral should be through (or with the support of) the GP. Supportive collaboration between primary and secondary health care teams is both good practice and a clinical necessity with such problems. This should be actively sought if necessary, especially when social services/Community Care Act assessment suggests it is appropriate, although urgent or special circumstances may require different approaches. Cases in secondary care may require direct specialist referral	NG	As above

Decision-making

Grading	Evidence suggests that:	Type	Source
	The individual with Alzheimer's disease and a designated decision-maker should have maximum involvement when decisions about the person with Alzheimer's disease are taking place. • The designated decision-maker should be an individual who can act in the best interests of the individual with Alzheimer's disease. • The designated decision-maker and the individual, if capable, should participate in decisions about personal and medical care participation in research, financial matters and place of residence. • The designated decision-maker should take into consideration any previously expressed wishes and demonstrated preferences of the individual.	NG	Alzheimer Society of Canada, 1992

Joint working

Grading	Evidence suggests that:	Type	Source
	It is important that easy referral between the old age psychiatry and the geriatric medical services is established. Often services facilitate this thorough regular joint clinical or educational activities.	NG	RCPsych, 1995

Organisation of care

Confidentiality

Grading	Evidence suggests that:	Type	Source
	Mandatory physician reporting of an Alzheimer's disease diagnosis (as exists in some states) compromises confidentiality.	NG	*ACCG, 1997b (from Post & Whitehouse, 1995)*

Communication

Grading	Evidence suggests that:	Type	Source
	Good communication with all involved is essential, not least with patient and carer. Specific team members (usually community psychiatric nurses or social workers) will routinely liaise with primary health care teams, social services/voluntary or private agencies. Written communication with the referring doctor is generally provided within a week of initial assessment, although more urgent telephone communication may also be necessary.	NG	*RCPsych, 1995*

Service provision (a) Case management

Grading	Evidence suggests that:	Type	Source
**	Studies of the effectiveness and efficiency of the case management approach are few and give inconclusive and contradictory results. One study suggested that individually tailored packages of care reduced the hospital admission rate, although this finding is not specific to people with dementia. This approach appears useful for the management of complex care needs. Like community resource teams, there is much research in this area at present and evaluation is not yet complete.	EBIP	*Melzer et al, 1994*

Service provision (b) Care planning

Grading	Evidence suggests that:	Type	Source
**	An individualised and comprehensive care plan should be prepared for each individual. The care plan should: • be based on the results of the assessment; • be designed to promote independence and maintain individuals at their maximum level of functioning; • deal with overall routine, behaviours, special activities and the social context of living; • offer the maximum degree of individualisation to accommodate the lifestyle, preferences, needs and strengths of the person with Alzheimer's disease and of the care-givers; and • be reviewed and updated by the inter-disciplinary team at least every four months.	NG	*Alzheimer Society of Canada, 1992*

Service provision (a) Care planning (continued)

Grading	Evidence suggests that:	Type	Source
	Care planning for the individual with Alzheimer's disease should be carried out by an inter-disciplinary team. • A basic team should consist of a family member and the paid care-giver with primary responsibility for providing direct care, plus other care providers as appropriate. • The individual's physician should be encouraged to play an active role in care and care planning should be included in team meetings. • The individual with Alzheimer's disease should be included as part of the team and should attend team meetings as appropriate.	NG	Alzheimer Society of Canada, 1992

Service provision (c) Community resource teams

Grading	Evidence suggests that:	Type	Source
**	Community resource teams (CRTs) attempt to provide flexible, tailored care across a range of services by assessing each dementia sufferer and carer needs in terms of mental, physical and social functioning. Requirements are reviewed repeatedly to ensure that care provision remains optimal throughout the course of the illness. CRTs are one example of the trend towards the integrated care approach. Studies to date on the effectiveness and efficiency of CRTs are few, inconclusive and sometimes contradictory. These studies suggest that this approach may initially result in an increase in admission rate in those living alone. Evaluation is not yet complete and this method of organisation of care deserves further development and testing.	EBIP	Melzer et al, 1994

Service provision (d) Special care units

Grading	Evidence suggests that:	Type	Source
*	Special care units may offer a model of optimal care for patients with dementia, although there is no evidence that special care units achieve better outcomes than traditional units.	EBG	APA, 1997

Organisation of care

Service provision (e) Residential care

Grading	Evidence suggests that:	Type	Source
***	A large number and proportion of nursing home residents in the US have dementia. Special care units are proliferating in response to concerns about the quality and appropriateness of the care they receive in most nursing homes. Experts in dementia care agree about the principles of care, but there is considerable disagreement about how the principles should be implemented, and existing special care units vary greatly in every respect. Evaluative research is needed to determine the impact of special care units on residents, families, staff members and nursing home residents without dementia. It is too soon for special regulations for special care units, but families and others need information about special care units to help them make decisions about placement of the person with dementia. Disclosure requirements are preferable to special regulations to protect patients and families from nursing homes that claim to provide special care but actually provide nothing special for their residents with dementia.	HTA	HTA Database; NHS CRD, 1998e (from Office of Technology Assessment, 1992)
***	Primary health care professionals should consider the use of structured programmes to encourage continuing independence for people with dementia resident in nursing homes.	EBG	CHSR, 1998
**	Health and social care professionals should be aware that the patient should not be assessed for optimal home care independently of the carer.	EBG	As above
**	Health and social care professionals should be aware that the following factors are known to increase the likelihood of people with dementia having to leave their own homes: carer stress, physical dependence, irritability, nocturnal wandering and incontinence.	EBG	As above
	Older adults worked through three phases as they made the initial transition to permanent residence in a nursing home.	CARS	*EBN*, 1998b (from Wilson, 1997)
	Care-giver training delayed admission of patients to nursing homes.	CARS	*EBMH*, 1998a (from Brodaty et al, 1997)
	The authors tried to ascertain the cost-per-QALY (quality-adjusted life-year) of group living compared with home living and residential care and compared with a combination of home and institutional care. The study does indicate that group living is a viable alternative to home and/or institutional living for patients with dementia but indicates even more strongly the need for further work into the quality of life associated with each of these residence regimes. (The NHS Centre for Reviews and Dissemination database includes a commentary. Users of this information are strongly advised to look this up before altering their practice).	EE	NEED; NHS CRD, 1998d (from Svensson et al, 1996)
	Many patients with dementia eventually require placement in a nursing home or other long-term care facility, and approximately two-thirds of nursing home patients suffer from dementia.	EBG	APA, 1997

Service provision (f) Primary care

Grading	Evidence suggests that:	Type	Source
**	GPs should consider the use of formal cognitive testing to enhance their clinical judgement.	EBG	CHSR, 1998
	GPs should, wherever possible, resist the routine use of tranquillisers to control behaviour disorders in patients with dementia.	EBG	As above
	Positive steps include the following: • Exclude treatable causes (in approximately 10%). • Exclude overlapping conditions e.g. depression, acute confusional state and psychotic symptoms, and concurrent physical illnesses. • Minimise associated disabilities. • Refer to consultant colleagues if the diagnosis is in doubt or to access additional resources. • Act as the gateway to other resources. • Help carers to care. Provide information and advice, especially about the emotional and behavioural changes which have already taken or will take place as the illness progresses. • Direct people to Alzheimer's Disease Society or Alzheimer Scotland – Action on Dementia.	NG	Alzheimer's Disease Society, 1995

Environment

Grading	Evidence suggests that:	Type	Source
***	Facilities should be structured to meet the needs of patients with dementia, including those with behavioural problems, which are extremely common.	EBG	APA, 1997
	The environment should reduce the confusion of the person with Alzheimer's disease. • The environment should convey a sense of familiarity to its users. • Areas should be laid out in a clear and well-ordered manner. • The environment should compensate for cognitive and perceptual deficits associated with Alzheimer's disease. • Whenever possible, there should be permanently designated areas for specific activities. • Visual and auditory stimulation should be at an appropriate level for the person with Alzheimer's disease.	NG	Alzheimer Society of Canada, 1992
	The environment should contribute to the effective functioning of the individual with Alzheimer's disease and their care-givers. • The environment should be designed to facilitate the variety of activities which will take place within the setting. • The environment should contain adequate space for freedom of mobility, including space to accommodate pacing. • The setting should be home-like and provide an acceptable level of privacy. • A separate space should be available to support the care-givers' need for privacy and respite.	NG	As above

Organisation of care

Environment (continued)

Grading	Evidence suggests that:	Type	Source
	The environment should meet the safety and security needs of the individual with Alzheimer's disease. • Individuals should be protected from hazards such as medications, poisonous materials, sharp objects, burns, falls and accidents. • The environment should be designed to allow individuals to wander safely. • Individuals should have access to secured outdoor space.	NG	Alzheimer Society of Canada, 1992

Transportation

Grading	Evidence suggests that:	Type	Source
	Vehicular transportation should be provided in a manner which ensures the safety and emotional comfort of the person with Alzheimer's disease. • Whenever possible, the driver should be accompanied by another individual. • The companion should be responsible for the safety of the passenger and for providing emotional support and assurance. • The companion should be aware of safety measures and the specific needs of the person with Alzheimer's disease. • The passenger should be accompanied to and from the vehicle. • Whenever possible, the travel time should be limited to the comfort level of the passenger.	NG	Alzheimer Society of Canada, 1992

Staff management

Grading	Evidence suggests that:	Type	Source
**	Staff with knowledge and experience concerning dementia and the management of non-cognitive symptoms appear to be important.	EBG	APA, 1997
	Health care professionals should be aware that the care setting and the attitudes of carers (or care teams in an institutional setting) may influence the emergence of behavioural problems.	EBG	CHSR, 1998
	An orientation program should be provided for all care-givers involved in services for people with Alzheimer's disease. • Staff and volunteers should receive an orientation to the facility or agency and to the programme for people with Alzheimer's disease. • Family members should receive an orientation to a setting or programme when their relative is admitted.	NG	Alzheimer Society of Canada, 1992
	All care-givers should have access to training and education which will help them understand the disease process and assist them in their role as care-giver: (a) formal and self-directed educational opportunities should be available for all care-givers; and (b) all care-givers should have access to a resource centre with current information on Alzheimer's disease and effective care-giving.	NG	As above

Staff management (continued)

Grading	Evidence suggests that:	Type	Source
	Performance appraisals should address the special issues facing staff and volunteers who provide care for people with Alzheimer's disease. • Performance appraisals for staff should be based on the extent to which they enhance the individual's dignity and autonomy, as well as their implementation of the individual care plan. • Performance appraisals for agency management should be based on their progress in achieving or exceeding the (Alzheimer Society of Canada's) guidelines for care. • Performance appraisals for volunteers should be based on their ability to effectively relate to the person with Alzheimer's disease.	NG	Alzheimer Society of Canada, 1992
	Procedures relating to the use of staff and volunteers in facilities and agencies should reflect the special requirements of people with Alzheimer's disease. • Staff and volunteers should be knowledgeable and skilled in providing care for people with Alzheimer's disease. • Wherever possible, staff and volunteers should have a previous record of working well with people with Alzheimer's disease. • Staff and volunteers should have chosen to work with people with Alzheimer's disease. • Continuity of staff and volunteers should be implemented to the fullest extent possible.	NG	As above
	Staff of facilities and agencies should be required to participate in a training and education program on meeting the needs of people with Alzheimer's disease and their care-givers. • The training and education programme should address information on Alzheimer's disease and should convey the knowledge and skills required to provide effective care. • The programme should deal with the motivational and psychosocial needs of individuals caring for people with Alzheimer's disease. • Staff of facilities and agencies should be trained on how to counsel, assist and communicate with family care-givers.	NG	As above

Learning disabilities and dementia

General

Grading	Evidence suggests that:	Type	Source
	Instituting medical and care management: Contact should be routine and ongoing between the paths of medical management (treatment of all treatable medical conditions, attention to coexisting mental disorders, frequent review of all medications with use of the fewest number and lowest possible doses, intensive care and deterrence of infection) and care management (documenting and implementing a treatment strategy appropriate to each stage of the disease, ensuring safety and a feeling of security in the environment, integration of family, friends, and companions into the overall care).	NG	Janicki et al, 1995 (American Association on Mental Retardation)

Learning disabilities

General (continued)

Grading	Evidence suggests that:	Type	Source
	Adults with learning disabilities who are at risk of Alzheimer's disease include those over the age of 50 years, those with Down's syndrome over the age of 40 years, or those who are from families with a history of Alzheimer's disease. The presence of any of these factors does not necessarily mean that dementia of the Alzheimer's type (or some other form of dementia) will occur. However, the presence of one or more of these risk factors may indicate an increased risk of an adult with learning disabilities developing this disease.	NG	Janicki *et al*, 1995 (American Association on Mental Retardation)
	Periodic screenings help identify potential changes in behaviour that may be indicative of pathological ageing. Changes that may be early indicators include: unexpected changes in routine behaviours; a decrement in functional abilities such as cooking, dressing or washing; memory losses or difficulty in learning new activities; changes in affect, attitude or demeanour; a loss of job or social skills; withdrawal from pleasurable activities; night-time awakenings and other altered time difficulties (temporal orientation); increase or decrease in rigid behavioural patterns; and onset of seizures. Because observable changes in behaviour may be due to causes other than dementia (e.g. depression, sensory impairments, hypo/hyperthyroidism) and may be treatable and reversible, referral for a diagnostic work-up should be made as soon as possible after observing any of the signs noted above.	NG	As above
	Further guidelines on the care of people with learning disabilities who have Alzheimer's disease are provided. The guidelines are very similar to those for people without learning disabilities. There is not space in this EBB to repeat the guidelines, but they can be obtained free of charge from the American Association on Mental Retardation – address supplied in Chapter 5.	NG	As above
	Although the staging of dementia symptoms does not appear to differ among people with learning disabilities in general, the manner in which symptoms may be expressed can vary widely from individual to individual. These symptoms may also appear differently among adults with Down's syndrome than among adults with other types of learning disability. For example, at the early stage of the disease among adults with Down's syndrome, memory loss is not always the first symptom noted and some symptoms ordinarily associated with onset of dementia of the Alzheimer's type may not occur. What may be observed are the following: an onset of seizures not previously observed, changes in personality, apathy, loss of conversational skills, possible incontinence and loss of self-care skills.	NG	As above
	It is advisable to conduct a baseline screening that includes cognitive, health and functional assessments beginning at the age of 40 in individuals at increased risk for premature ageing, such as persons with Down's syndrome, and beginning at the age of 50 in others. Following this, the individual should receive periodic cognitive, health and functional assessments that reveal significant changes in function.	NG	As above

General *(continued)*

Grading	Evidence suggests that:	Type	Source
	The diagnostic evaluation should also include a thorough physical and neurological examination, including the testing of sensory-motor systems (especially visual and hearing problems) to rule out other disorders. A mental status test may be used as a quick means to screen for problems in orientation, attention, recent recall and the ability (as appropriate to learning level) to calculate, read, write, name, copy a drawing, repeat, understand and make judgements. Mental status examinations, however, may give little information on individuals with severe cognitive limitations. In these situations, mental status examinations need to take into account the individual's past history and abilities and should never be used as the sole clinical assessment.	NG	Janicki *et al*, 1995 (American Association on Mental Retardation)
	When there is suspicion of the presence of dementia of the Alzheimer's type, referral for a thorough evaluation should be made to assure a proper differential diagnosis. Respond to noticed changes by: • gathering information on behaviour to further confirm noticed changes, preferably from multiple informants such as staff or carers; • continuing to monitor behaviour/function to have complete information for clinicians; and • making referral for a diagnostic work-up for the purpose of a differential diagnosis. To make a distinction between possible and probable diagnosis of Alzheimer's disease, it is necessary to observe a well-documented progression of symptoms substantiated by appropriate clinical test results. Because periodic observation of behaviour is one of the critical features of a diagnostic evaluation among adults with learning disabilities, obtaining a confident diagnosis will require repeated evaluations.	NG	As above
	A complete diagnostic evaluation should include a detailed medical history, provided by a family member, carer or someone else well-acquainted with the individual. The medical history should include medication use, past and present illnesses, previous treatments, hospitalisations and family history of dementia. This is to accurately determine whether or not there has been progressive deterioration of skills and noticeable personality changes, problems with memory and difficulty with daily activities. As much as possible, the adult with learning disabilities should be involved in this process and asked what he or she feels is different or changing. For persons with Down's or Prader–Willi syndrome, assessment should also look for signs of sleep apnoea.	NG	As above
	A periodically applied screening instrument should be used to establish both a behavioural baseline and to obtain longitudinal measures that indicate change. Where periodic screenings are not practical or possible, an alternative means of assessing change may be accomplished by having the individual keep a life-history record in which are noted significant events, abilities and documentation of other capabilities. Such baseline measures or life-histories permit an understanding of normative behaviour and highlight the significance of any changes that indicate possible pathological ageing. Indications of change may also come from comprehensive geriatric assessments, primary care screenings (e.g. thyroid, hearing, vision tests) and cognitive or functional assessments.	NG	As above

Learning disabilities

References

Abstracts of Clinical Care Guidelines (funded by the National Study Group, National Genome Research Institute of the National Institute of Health) (1997a) *Abstracts of Clinical Care Guidelines*, **9**, 19–20. Abstract of: Post, S., Whitehouse, P., instock, R., *et al* (1997) The clinical introduction of genetic testing for Alzheimer disease. *Journal of the American Medical Association,* **277**, 832–836.

Abstracts of Clinical Care Guidelines (funded by the Cleveland Community Dialogue on Ethics and the Progression of Dementia (1997b) *Abstracts of Clinical Care Guidelines*, **9**, 21–22. Abstract of: Post, S. & Whitehouse, P. (1995) Fairhill guidelines on ethics of the care of people with Alzheimer's disease: a clinical summary. *Journal of the American Geriatrics Society,* **43**, 1423–1429.

ACP Journal Club (1991a) Dementia severity, wandering and falling, and behavioral problems were associated with shorter survival in Alzheimer disease. *ACP Journal Club,* **114**, 21. Abstract of: Walsh J. S., Welch G. & Larson E. B. (1990) Survival of outpatients with Alzheimer-type dementia. *Annals of Internal Medicine,* **113**, 429–434.

—— (1991b) Intramuscular desferrioxamine slowed the decline in living skills in Alzheimer disease. *ACP Journal Club,* **115**, 41. Abstract of: McLachlan D., Dalton A., Kruck T., *et al* (1991) Intramuscular desferrioxamine in patients with Alzheimer's disease. *Lancet.* **337**, 1304–1308.

—— (1991c) Review: Test characteristics and pretest probability of disease need to be considered in screening for dementia. *ACP Journal Club,* **115**, 88. Abstract of: Siu, A. L. (1991) Screening for dementia and investigating its causes. *Annals of Internal Medicine,* **15**, 122–132.

—— (1991d) Triazolam caused sedation and impairment of psychomotor performance in elderly persons. *ACP Journal Club,* **115**, 94. Revised 1996. Abstract of: Greenblatt, D., Harmatz, J S., Shapiro, L., *et al* (1991) Sensitivity to triazolam in the elderly. *New England Journal of Medicine,* **324**, 1691–1698.

—— (1992) 12-month trial of acetyl-L-carnitine for Alzheimer's disease. *ACP Journal Club,* **116**, 81. Abstract of: Spagnoli, A., Lucca, U., Menasce, G., *et al* (1991) Long-term acetyl-L-carnitine treatment in Alzheimer's disease. *Neurology,* **41**, 1726–32.

—— (1994) High-dose tacrine improved symptoms in patients with Alzheimer disease. *ACP Journal Club,* **121**, 37. Abstract of: Knapp, M. J., Knopman, D. S., Solomon P. R., *et al* (1994) A 30-week randomized controlled trial of high-dose tacrine in patients with Alzheimer's disease. *Journal of the American Medical Association,* **271**, 985–991.

—— (1995) Hydergine is effective for dementia. *ACP Journal Club,* **122**, 17. Abstract of: Schneider, L. S. & Olin, J. T. (1994) Overview of clinical trials of hydergine in dementia. *Archives of Neurology,* **51**, 787–798.

—— (1997a) Algorithms provided useful information about the course of Alzheimer disease. *ACP Journal Club,* **127**, 43. Abstract of: Stern, Y., Tang, M. X., Albert, M. S., *et al* (1997) Predicting time to nursing home care and death in individuals with Alzheimer disease. *Journal of the American Medical Association,* **277**, 806–812.

—— (1997b) NSAIDs but not aspirin or acetaminophen reduced the risk for Alzheimer disease *ACP Journal Club,* **127**, 46. Abstract of: Stewart, W. F., Kawas, C., Corrada, M., *et al* (1997) Risk of Alzheimer's disease and duration of NSAID use. *Neurology,* **48**, 626–632.

Agency for Health Care Policy and Research (AHCPR) (1996) *Recognition and Initial Assessment of Alzheimer's Disease and Related Dementias: Clinical Practice Guideline No. 19,* pp. 1–143. Rockville, MD: AHCPR.

Alzheimer Society of Canada (1992) *Guidelines for Care,* pp. 1–27. Toronto: Alzheimer Society of Canada.

Alzheimer's Disease Society. (1995) *Dementia in the Community: Management Strategies for General Practice,* pp. 1–34. London: Alzheimer's Disease Society.

American Academy of Neurology (Quality Standards Subcommittee) (1994) Practice parameter for diagnosis and evaluation of dementia. *Neurology,* **44,** 2203–2206.

American Psychiatric Association (1997) Practice guidelines for the treatment of patients with Alzheimer's disease and other dementias of later life. *American Journal of Psychiatry,* **154,** 1–39.

Bandolier (1995) Falls in the elderly. *Bandolier,* **3,** 3.

Bandolier (1997) New dementia drug. *Bandolier,* **4,** 2–3.

Bandolier (1998) Dementia – diagnosis and treatment. *Bandolier,* **5,** 2–3.

Birks, J. & Flicker, L. (1998) *The Efficacy and Safety of Selegiline for the Symptomatic Treatment of Alzheimer's Disease: A Systematic Review of the Evidence.* In: the Cochrane Library. Oxford: Update Software Ltd.

Bowling, A., Grundy, E. & Farquhar, M. (1997) Living well into old age. In *Social Care Research.* Report No. 5, pp. 1–5. York: Joseph Rowntree Foundation.

Britton, A. & Russell, R. (1998) *Multidisciplinary Team Interventions in the Management of Delirium in Patients with Chronic Cognitive Impairment – A Review of the Evidence of Effectiveness.* In: the Cochrane Library. Oxford: Update Software Ltd.

Centre for Evidence-Based Medicine (CEBM) (1997) Alzheimer's disease – support for caregivers delayed time to nursing home placement. CAT Bank. Abstract of: Mittelman, M., Ferris, S. H., Shulman, E., *et al* (1996) A family intervention to delay nursing home placement of patients with Alzheimer's disease. *Journal of the American Medical Association,* **276,** 1725–1731.

Centre for Health Services Research and Department of Primary Care (CHSR) (1998) *The Primary Care Management of Dementia. North of England Evidence-Based Guideline Development Project,* pp. 1–98. Newcastle: CHSR.

Evidence-Based Medicine (1996) Moclobemide was an effective antidepressant in elderly patients with cognitive decline and depression. *Evidence-Based Medicine,* **1,** 202. Abstract of: Roth, M., Mountjoy, C., Amrein, R., *et al* (and the International Collaborative Study Group (1996) Moclobemide in elderly patients with cognitive decline and depression. An international double-blind, placebo-controlled trial. *British Journal of Psychiatry,* **168,** 149–157.

—— (1997*a*) Mini-Mental State Examination and the Informant Questionnaire on Cognitive Decline were efficient screening tests for dementia. *Evidence-Based Medicine,* **2,** 25. Abstract of: Mulligan, R., Mackinnon, A., Jorm, A. F., *et al* (1996) A comparison of alternative methods of screening for dementia in clinical settings. *Archives of Neurology,* **53,** 532–536.

—— (1997*b*) Post menopausal oestrogen reduced the risk for and delayed the onset of Alzheimer disease. *Evidence-Based Medicine,* **2,** 28. Abstract of: Tang, M., Jacobs, D., Stern, Y., *et al* (1996) Effect of oestrogen during menopause on risk and age at onset of Alzheimer's disease. *Lancet,* **348,** 429–432.

—— (1997*c*) Support for caregivers delayed time to nursing home placement in Alzheimer's disease. *Evidence-Based Medicine,* **2,** 85. Abstract of: Mittelman, M., Ferris, S. H., Shulman, E., *et al* (1996) A family intervention to delay nursing home placement of patients with Alzheimer disease. A randomized controlled trial. *Journal of the American Medical Association,* **276,** 1725–1731.

—— (1997*d*) Selegiline, or alpha-tocopherol, slowed the progression of Alzheimer disease. *Evidence-Based Medicine,* **2**, 175. Abstract of: Sano, M., Ernesto, C., Thomas, R. G., *et al* (for the members of the Alzheimer's Disease Cooperative Study) (1997) A controlled trial of selegiline, alpha-tocopherol, or both as a treatment for Alzheimer's disease. *New England Journal of Medicine*, **336**, 1216–1222.

—— (1997*e*) Driving cessation was associated with depressive symptoms among older persons. *Evidence-Based Medicine,* **2**, 176. Abstract of: Marattoli, R. A., Mendes de Leon, C. F., Glass, T. A., *et al* (1997) Driving cessation and increased depressive symptoms: Prospective evidence from the New Haven EPESE. *Journal of the American Geriatric Society*, **45**, 202–206.

—— (1998) Gingko biloba safely and modestly improved dementia. *Evidence-Based Medicine,* **3**, 81. Abstract of: Le Bars, P. L., Katz, M. M, Berman, N., *et al* (for the North American Evidence BasedStudy Group) (1997) A placebo controlled double blind randomised trial of an extract of Ginkgo biloba for dementia. *Journal of the American Medical Association*, **278**, 1327–1333.

Evidence-Based Mental Health (1998*a*) Caregiver training delayed admission of patients with dementia to nursing homes. *Evidence-Based Mental Health,* **1**, 9. Abstract of: Brodaty, H., Gresham, M. & Luscombe, G. (1997) The Prince Henry Hospital dementia caregivers' training programme. *International Journal of Geriatric Psychiatry*, **12**, 183–192.

—— (1998*b*) Donepezil improved cognitive and global function in mild to moderate Alzheimer's disease. *Evidence-Based Mental Health,* **1**, 88. Abstract of: Rogers S. L., Farlow M. R., Doody R. S., *et al* (1998) A 24-week, double-blind, placebo-controlled trial of donepezil in patients with Alzheimer's disease. *Neurology*, **50**, 136–145.

Evidence-Based Nursing (1998*a*) A risk assessment score predicted which elderly patients would fall during a hospital stay. *Evidence-Based Nursing,* **1**, 89. Abstract of: Oliver, D., Britton, M., Seed, P., *et al* (1997) Development and evaluation of an evidence-based risk assessment tool (STRATIFY) to predict which elderly in-patients will fall: case control and cohort studies. *British Medical Journal*, **315**, 1049–1053.

—— (1998*b*) Older adults worked through 3 phases as they made the initial transition to permanent residence in a nursing home. *Evidence-Based Nursing,* **1**, 96. Abstract of: Wilson, S. A. (1997) The transition to nursing home life: a comparison of planned and unplanned admission. *Journal of Advanced Nursing*, **26**, 867–871.

Fioravanti, M. & Yanagi, M. (1998) *CDP-Choline in the Treatment of Cognitive and Behavioural Disturbances Associated with Chronic Cerebral Disorders of the Aged.* In: the Cochrane Library. Oxford: Update Software Ltd.

Flicker, L. & Grimley-Evans, J. (1998) *The Efficacy of Piracetam in Patients with Dementia or Cognitive Impairment.* In: the Cochrane Library. Oxford: Update Software Ltd.

Folstein, M. F., Folstein, S. E., McHugh, P. R. (1975) Mini-Mental State: a practical method for grading the cognitive state of patients for the clinician. *Journal of Psychiatric Research*, **12**, 196–198.

Haines, A. & Katona, C. (1992) Dementia in old age. In *Clinical Guidelines: Occasional Paper Number 58* pp. 62–66. London: Royal College of General Practitioners.

Higgins, J. & Flicker, L. (1998) *The Efficacy of Lecithin in the Treatment of Dementia and Cognitive Impairment.* In: the Cochrane Library. Oxford: Update Software Ltd.

Hodkinson, H. M. (1972) Evaluation of a mental test score for assessment of mental impairment in the elderly. *Age and Ageing*, **1**, 233–238.

Huppert, F., Van Niekerk, J., Herbert, J. (1998) *The Effect of DHEA Supplementation in Well-Being and Cognition.* In: the Cochrane Library. Oxford: Update Software Ltd.

Janicki, M., Heller, T., Selzer, G., et al (1995) *Practice guideline for the clinical assessment and care management of Alzheimer and other dementias among adults with mental retardation: Report of the AAMR–IASSID Work group on Practice Guidelines for the Care Management of Alzheimer's Disease.* Washingon, DC: American Association on Mental Retardation.

Journal of Evidence-Based Practice POEM (1997a) Donepezil for Alzheimer's disease. *Journal of Evidence-Based Practice POEM.* Abstract of: Rogers S. L., Farlow M. R., Doody R. S., et al (1998) A 24-week, double-blind, placebo-controlled trial of donepezil in patients with Alzheimer's disease. *Neurology*, **50**, 136–145.

—— (1997b) Gingko biloba for dementia. *Journal of Evidence-Based Practice* POEM. Abstract of: Le Bars, P. L., Katz, M. M., Berman, N., et al (for the North American Evidence Based Study Group) (1997) A placebo-controlled, double-blind, randomized trial of an extract of Gingko biloba for dementia. *Journal of the American Medical Association*, **278**, 1327–1332.

—— (1997c) Selegiline and vitamin E in Alzheimer's disease. *Journal of Evidence-Based Practice* POEM. Abstract of: Sano, M., Ernesto, C., Thomas, R. G. (1997) *New England Journal of Medicine*, **336**, 1216.

Katzman, R., Brown, T., Fuld, P, et al (1983) Validation of a short orientation-memory concentration test of cognitive impairment. *American Journal of Psychiatry*, **140**, 734–739.

Kokmen, E., Naessens, J. M. & Offord, K. P. (1987) A short test of mental status: description and preliminary results. *Mayo Clinic Procedures*, **62**, 281–288.

Melzer, D., Hopkins, S., Pencheon, D., et al (1994) Dementia. In *Health Care Needs Assessment: The Epidemiologically Based Needs Assessment Reviews*, pp. 303–340. Oxford: Radcliffe Medical Press.

NHS Centre for Reviews and Dissemination (1998a) Confused Minds, Burdened Families: Finding Help for People with Alzheimer's and Other Dementias. Health Technology Assessment Database. Abstract of: Office of Technology Assessment (1990) *Confused Minds, Burdened Families: Finding Help for People with Alzheimer's and Other Dementias*, p. 424. Washington DC: US Congress.

—— (1998b) *Differentiation of Dementia and Depression by Memory Tests: A Meta-Analysis.* Database of Abstract Reviews of Effectiveness (DARE). In: the Cochrane Library. Oxford: Update Software Ltd. Abstract of: Lachner, G. & Engel, R. R. (1994) Differentiation of dementia and depression by memory tests: a meta-analysis. *Journal of Nervous and Mental Disease*, **182**, 34–39.

(1998c) Economic evaluation of a support program for caregivers of demented elderly. NHS Economic Evaluation Database (NEED). Abstract of: Drummond, M. F., Mohide, E. A., Tew, M., et al (1991) Economic evaluation of a support program for caregivers of demented elderly. *International Journal of Technology Assessment in Health Care*, **7**, 209–219.

—— (1998d) Group living for elderly patients with dementia: a cost analysis. NHS Economic Evaluation Database (NEED). Abstract of: Svensson, M., Edebalk, P. G. & Persson, U. (1996) Group living for elderly patients with dementia: a cost analysis. *Health Policy*, **38**, 83–100.

—— (1998e) Special Care Units for People with Alzheimer's and Other Dementias: Consumer Education, Research, Regulatory and Reimbursement Issues. Health Technology Assessment Database. Abstract of: Office of Technology Assessment (1992) *Special Care Units for People with Alzheimer's and Other Dementias: Consumer Education, Research, Regulatory and Reimbursement Issues*, p. 204. Washington DC: US Congress.

—— (1998f) The costs and benefits of a screening program to detect dementia in older drivers. NHS Economic Evaluation Database (NEED). Abstract of: Retchin, S. M. & Hillner, B. E. (1994) The costs and benefits of a screening program to detect dementia in older drivers. *Medical Decision Making*, **14**, 315–324.

—— (1998g) *The Effect of Therapy on the Mental Health of the Elderly*. Database of Abstract Reviews of Effectiveness (DARE). In: the Cochrane Library. Oxford: Update Software Ltd. Abstract of: Burckhardt, C. (1987) The effect of therapy on the mental health of the elderly. *Research in Nursing & Health*, **10**, 277–285.

—— (1998h) Selegiline in treatment of behavioural and cognitive symptoms of Alzheimer disease. Database of Abstract Reviews of Effectiveness (DARE). *Cochrane Library*, Issue 3. Abstract of: Tolbert, S. R. & Fuller, M. A. (1996) Selegiline in the treatment of behavioral and cognitive symptoms of Alzheimer disease. *Annals of Pharmacotherapy*, **30**, 1122–1129.

—— & Nuffield Institute for Health (1996) Preventing falls and subsequent injury in older people. *Effective Health Care*, **2**, 1.

Olin, J., Schneider, L., Novit, A., *et al* (1998) Efficacy of Hydergine for Dementia. In: the Cochrane Library. Oxford: Update Software Ltd.

Pattie, A. H. & Gilleard, C. J. (1975) A brief psychogeriatric assessment schedule. Validation against psychiatric diagnosis and discharge from hospital. *British Journal of Psychiatry*, **127**, 489–493.

Pfeffer, R. I., Kursaki, T. T., Harrah, C. H., *et al* (1982) Measurement of functional activities of older adults in the community. *Journal of Gerontology*, **37**, 232–329.

Qizilbash, N., Birks, J., Lopez Arrieta, J., et al (1998a) *The Efficacy of Tacrine in Alzheimer's Disease*. In: the Cochrane Library. Oxford: Update Software Ltd.

——, Lopez Arrieta, J. & Birks, J. (1998b) *Nimodipine in the Treatment of Primary Degenerative, Mixed and Vascular Dementia*. In: the Cochrane Library. Oxford: Update Software Ltd.

Royal College of Psychiatrists (1995) *Consensus Statement on the Assessment and Investigation of an Elderly Person with Suspected Cognitive Iimpairment by a Specialist Old Age Psychiatry Service*. Council Report CR49. London: Royal College of Psychiatrists.

Scottish Intercollegiate Guidelines Network (SIGN) (1998) *Interventions in the Management of Behavioural and Psychological Aspects of Dementia*. SIGN Publication No. 22. Edinburgh: SIGN.

Standing Medical Advisory Committee (1998) *The Use of Donepezil for Alzheimer's Disease*, p. 1. London: Department of Health.

Spector, A. & Orrell, M. (1998a) *Reminiscence Therapy for Dementia: A Review of the Evidence of Effectiveness*. In: the Cochrane Library. Oxford: Update Software Ltd.

—— & —— (1998b) *Reality orientation for dementia: a review of the evidence of effectiveness*. In: the Cochrane Library. Oxford: Update Software Ltd.

Stein, K. (1997) *Donezepil in the treatment of mild to moderate senile dementia of the Alzheimer type (SDAT)*. NHSE South & West R & D: Wessex Insititute.

Thompson, C. & Thompson, G. (1998) Support for carers of people with Alzheimer's type dementia. In: the Cochrane Library. Oxford: Update Software Ltd.

US Department of Veterans Affairs & University Health System Consortium (1997) *Dementia Identification and Assessment: Guidelines for Primary Care Practitioners*. IL: Oak Brook.

US Preventive Services Task Force (1996) *Screening for Dementia*, pp. 531–540. Baltimore, MA: Williams & Wilkins.

4. Critical appraisal tools

Introduction

This chapter provides two critical appraisal tools:

(1) Critical appraisal form for an overview: use this form to appraise systematic reviews, meta-analyses and other overviews.

(2) Critical appraisal form for clinical guidelines: use this form to appraise clinical practice guidelines.

N.B. Both of these forms may be photocopied freely.

It is recommended that EBB users obtain the full version of the sources used in this EBB. Chapter 5 provides details on how to obtain this information. The evidence can then be appraised using one of the two appraisal tools provided in this chapter.

This chapter ends by providing details on how to obtain further critical appraisal tools which can be used for other types of research evidence.

Critical appraisal tool 1

Critical appraisal form for an overview

(adapted from material produced by the Centre for Evidence-Based Mental Health)

Title of paper . . . .

Author . . . .

Source . . . .

Date . . . .

Are the results valid?	Y	N	*Comments*
(1) Did the review address select a clearly focused issue? Did the review describe: • the population studied? • the intervention given? • the outcomes considered?			
(2) Did the authors select the right sort of studies for the review? The right studies would: • address the review's questions • have an adequate study design			
(3) Do you think the important, relevant studies were included? Look for: • which bibliographic databases were used • personal contact with experts • search for unpublished as well as published studies • search for non-English language studies			
(4) Did the review's authors do enough to assess the quality of the included studies? Did they use: • description of randomisation? • a rating scale?			

What are the results?	*Y*	*N*	*Comments*
(5) Were the results similar from study to study? Are the results of all the included studies clearly displayed? • Are the results from different studies similar? • If not, are the reasons for variations between the studies discussed?			
(6) What is the overall result of the review? Is there a clinical bottom-line? • What is it? • What is the numerical result?			
(7) How precise are the results? • Is there a confidence interval?			

Can I use the results to help my patients?	*Y*	*N*	*Comments*
(8) Can I apply the results to my patients? • Is this patient so different from those in the review that the results do not apply?			
(9) Should I apply the results to my patient? • How great would the benefit of therapy be for this particular patient? • Is the intervention consistent with my patient's values and preferences? • Were all the clinically important outcomes considered? • Do the benefits outweigh the harms and costs?			

Critical appraisal tool 2

Critical appraisal form for clinical guidelines
(adapted from material produced by the Centre for Evidence-Based Medicine)

Title of paper . . . .

Author . . . .

Source . . . .

Date . . . .

Are the recommendations in these guidelines valid?	*Y*	*N*	*Unclear*	*Page no.*
(1) Were all important decision options and outcomes clearly defined?				
(2) Was the evidence relevant to each decision option identified, validated and combined in a sensible and explicit way?				
(3) Are the relative preferences that key stakeholders attach to the outcomes of decisions (including benefits, risks and costs) identified and explicitly considered?				
(4) Are the guidelines resistant to clinically sensible variations in practice?				

Are these guidelines potentially useful?	*Y*	*N*	*Unclear*	*Page no.*
(5) Does this guideline offer an opportunity for significant improvement in the quality of health care practice?				
• Is there large variation in current practice?				
• Do these guidelines contain new evidence (or old evidence not yet acted upon) that could have an important impact on management?				
• Would these guidelines affect the management of so many people, or concern individuals at such high risk, or involve such high costs that even small changes in practice could have major impacts on health outcomes or resources?				

Should these guidelines be applied in your practice?	Y	N	Unclear	Comments
(6) Can any barriers to its implementation be overcome?				
(7) Can they be overcome?				
(8) Can you meet the variety of conditions which will determine the success or failure of implementing the guidelines? For example:				

- Has the evidence been collated by a respected body? (e.g. rigorously developed clinical practice guidelines from a Medical Royal College)

- Are local opinion leaders already implementing the strategy?

- Have you received consistent information from all sources?

- Has a 'user-friendly' format for the guidelines been developed (may require local adoption)?

- Can you implement the guidelines within a target group of clinicians (without the need for extensive outside collaboration?

- Do the guidelines represent a conflict of interest with patient and community expectations, economic incentives, administrative incentives, etc.?

Additional comments:

Resources for critical appraisal and systematic searching

Additional resources to support critical appraisal, systematic searching and developing structured questions are provided by the following organisations.

Centre for Evidence-Based Mental Health

The Centre for Evidence-Based Mental Health provides a tool kit of appraisal tools, clinical scenarios and teaching materials specifically developed for use in mental health services. The centre is currently compiling a database of critically appraised topics in mental health (the CAT Bank) and it also provides a comprehensive list of links to critical appraisal resources provided by other organisations.

The critical appraisal tools can be found on the internet at:

http://www.psychiatry.ox.ac.uk/cebmh/toolkit/appraising.html

Critical appraisal forms provided currently include those for:

- overviews
- single therapy studies
- diagnosis
- prognosis

Contact details:

Centre for Evidence-Based Mental Health
Department of Psychiatry
University of Oxford
Warneford Hospital
Oxford OX3 7LF
Tel: 01865 226480
Fax: 01865 793101
E-mail: cebmh.enquiries@psychiatry.ox.ac.uk
Website: www.psychiatry.ox.ac.uk/cebmh/

Centre for Evidence-Based Medicine

The Centre for Evidence-Based Medicine provides appraisal worksheets produced by Professor David Sackett. These can be accessed through the centre's website:

http://wwwcebm.jr2.ox.ac.uk/docs/teaching.html

Critical appraisal forms provided include those for:

- overview (of therapy)
- diagnosis
- prognosis
- harm/aetiology
- economic analysis
- decision analysis

The Centre for Evidence-Based Medicine also provides sample search strategies which can be accessed at:

http://cebm.jr2.ox.ac.uk/docs/searching.html

Contact details:

Centre for Evidence-Based Medicine
Nuffield Department of Clinical Medicine
Level 5, Oxford Radcliffe NHS Trust
Headley Way
Headington
Oxford OX3 9DU
Tel: 01865 741166
Website: cebm.jr2.ox.ac.uk/

Cochrane Collaboration

The Cochrane Collaboration Review Groups each produce standardised systematic search strategies.

Cochrane Review Groups relevant to this EBB include:

- Dementia and Cognitive Impairment
- Depression, Anxiety and Neurosis
- Drugs and Alcohol
- Consumers and Communication

The Cochrane Library includes details of these search strategies and is available from:

Update Software
PO Box 696
Oxford OX2 7YX
Tel: 01865 513902
Fax: 01865 516918
E-mail: update@cochrane.co.uk

http://update.cochrane.co.uk/info/

Training

The following organisations provide training events for evidence-based practice and critical appraisal:

Centre for Evidence-Based Mental Health and
Centre for Evidence-Based Medicine (details above)

Critical Appraisal Skills Programme (CASP)
Institute of Health Sciences
Anglia & Oxford Regional Health Authority
Old Road
Headington
Oxford OX3 7LF
Tel: 01865 226968
Fax: 01865 226775
E-mail: casp@cix.co.uk
Website: www.ihs.ox.ac.uk/casp/frameset.html

North Thames Research Appraisal Group
Royal Free School of Medicine
Department of Primary Care & Population Sciences
Upper 3rd Floor
Rowland Hill Street
London NW3 2PF
Tel: 0171 830 2549
Fax: 0171 794 1224
E-mail: ntrag@rfhsm.ac.uk
Website: cebm.jr2.ox.ac.uk/ntrag/ntrag.html

Useful references

Dixon R. A., Munro, J. F. & Silcocks P. B. (1997) *The Evidence-Based Medicine Workbook: Critical Appraisal for Problem Solving.* Oxford: Butterworth Heinemann.

Greenhalgh, T. (1997) *How to Read a Paper: The Basics of Evidence-Based Medicine.* London: BMJ Publishing Group.

Gray, J. A. M. (1997) *Evidence-Based Healthcare: How to Make Health Policy and Management Decision.* Edinburgh: Churchill Livingstone.

Sackett, D. L., Richardson, W. S., Rosenberg, W., *et al* (1997) *Evidence-Based Medicine: How to Practise and Teach EBM.* Churchill Livingstone, Edinburgh.

Sackett, D. L., Haynes, R. B., Guyatt, G. H., *et al* (1991) *Clinical Epidemiology: A Basic Science for Clinical Medicine (2nd Edition).* Boston, MA: Little Brown & Co.

Straus, S. E., Badenoch, D., Richardson, W. S., *et al* (1998) *Practising Evidence-Based Medicine: Tutor's Manual (3rd Edition).*Oxford: Radcliffe Medical Press Ltd.

5. Sources of information

EBB sources of evidence

We strongly recommend that you obtain the originals of the evidence included in this EBB. This chapter provides information about the providers of the information used in this EBB, along with their contact details.

Guidelines

Source	Remit of information source	Contact details
US Agency for Health Care Policy adn Research (AHCPR)	The AHCPR is an agency of the US Government's Department of Health and Human Services. Its remit is to enhance the quality, appropriateness and effectiveness of health care services and access to these services. It commissions guideline development panels which employ an explicit science-based methodology and expert clinical judgement to develop specific statements on patient assessment and management for the clinical condition selected.	AHCPR Publications Clearing House PO 8547 Silver Spring, MD 20907 Tel: 001-800-358-9295 E-mail: info@ahcpr.gov http://www.ahcpr.gov/
Scottish Inter-Collegiate Guidelines Network (SIGN)	SIGN is a network of clinicians and health care professionals. Its objective is to improve the effectiveness and efficiency of clinical care for patients in Scotland by developing, publishing and disseminating guidelines which identify and promote good clinical practice. SIGN has produced evidence-based national recommendations.	SIGN Royal College of Physicians of Edinburgh 9 Queen Street Edinburgh EH2 1JQ Tel: 0131 225 7324 Fax: 0131 225 1769 E-mail: r.harbour@rcpe.ac.uk http://pc47.cee.hw.ac.uk/sign
American Psychiatric Association (APA)	The APA is the professional body for psychiatry in the US. It produces reliable and valid guidelines consistent with the recommendations of the American Medical Association and the Institute of Medicine.	American Psychiatric Association 1400 K Street, N.W. Washington, DC *Available in the UK from:* American Psychiatric Press Inc. c/o Eurospan, 3 Henrietta Street London WC2E 8LU
The Royal College of Psychiatrists' (RCPsych) Research Unit	The Royal College of Psychiatrists' Research Unit undertakes a wide range of work related to clinical effectiveness. This includes an evidence-based guidelines development programme, guidelines in mental health, the production of evidence-base briefings, support for national multi-centre clinical audit projects and the development of outcome measures.	Sam Coombs Royal College of Psychiatrists' Research Unit 11 Grosvenor Crescent London SW1X 7EE Tel: 0171 235 2351, ext. 234 Fax: 0171 235 2954 E-mail: scoombs@rcpsych.ac.uk
RCPsych *Guidelines in Mental Health: A Bibliography*	*Guidelines in Mental Health* is a bibliography arranged into 25 subject headings, of national and international mental health guidelines, Cochrane Collaboration reviews and records from the Database of Abstracts of Reviews of Effectiveness.	Victoria Thomas Royal College of Psychiatrists' Research Unit 11 Grosvenor Crescent London SW1X 7EE Tel: 0171 235 2351, ext. 282 Fax: 0171 235 2954 E-mail: victoria.thomas@virgin.net

Guidelines (continued)

Source	Remit of information source	Contact details
RCPsych guidelines	The Royal College of Psychiatrists has an established programme of development of evidence-based guidelines. The following has been published: *Management of Imminent Violence: Clinical Practice Guidelines to Support Mental Health Services (Occasional Paper OP41). Management of Schizophrenia* will be the next in this series. These guidelines are also accessible through the Centre for Evidence-Based Mental Health website. http://www.psychiatry.ox.ac.uk/cebmh/	Available from: Book Sales Department Royal College of Psychiatrists 17 Belgrave Square London SW1X 7EE Tel: 0171 235 2351, ext. 146 Fax: 0171 235 1231 E-mail: booksales@rcpsych.ac.uk
RCPsych Library	The Royal College of Psychiatrists' Library holds an extensive collection of policy and guideline reports related to mental health and includes all Royal College of Psychiatrists publications. The library also performs CD-ROM searches on Medline and ClinPsyc.	The Librarian Royal College of Psychiatrists' Library 17 Belgrave Square London SW1X 8PG Tel: 0171 235 2351, ext. 138
Guideline	Guideline is a UK-based initiative to develop an electronic database of critically-appraised, clinical practice guidelines for health and allied care professionals across the NHS.	Project Officer Institute of Health Sciences Old Road, Headington Oxford OX3 7LF Tel: 01865 226607 Fax: 01865 226879 E-mail: ainglis@care.phru.org http://www.ihs.ox.ac.uk/ guidelines/index.html

Internet sites with searches and links to sites providing evidence-based information

Source	Remit of information source	Contact details
Centre for Evidence-Based Mental Health and OXAMWEB	The Centre produces a wide range of resources to support evidence-based practice in mental health, including critical appraisal tools, training, a collection of critically appraised topics (the CAT Bank), etc. It also manages the Oxford and Anglia Mental Health Web (OXAMWEB).	http://www.psychiatry.ox.ac.uk/cebmh/
Turning Research Into Practice (TRIP)	Oxamweb aims to provide all sorts of information (evidence-based, textbook style, etc.), within three clicks or fewer, to support evidence-based practice in mental health. Part of the Clinical Effectiveness Initiative for Wales, TRIP provides a facility for searching the internet sites of a wide range of providers of evidence-based information.	http://www.gwent.nhs.gov.uk/trip

Systematic reviews

Source	Remit of information source	Contact details
Cochrane Library	The Cochrane Collaboration is an international organisation that aims to help people make well-informed decisions about health care by preparing, maintaining and promoting the accessibility of systematic reviews of the effects of health care interventions. The Cochrane Collaboration produces the Cochrane Library which consists of the Cochrane Database of Systematic Reviews, Database of Abstracts of Reviews of Effectiveness, the Cochrane Controlled Trials Register and the Cochrane Review Methodology Database.	Cochrane Collaboration Secretariat PO Box 726, Oxford OX2 7UX Tel: 01865 310138 Fax: 01865 516311 E-mail: secretariat@cochrane.co.uk *Cochrane Library orders:* Update Software Ltd. Summertown Pavilion Middle Way, Oxford OX2 7LG Tel: 01865 513902 Fax: 01865 516918 E-mail: sales@update.co.uk http://www.cochrane.co.uk
NHS Centre for Reviews & Dissemination (NHS CRD)	The NHS CRD is funded by the NHS Executive to produce systematic reviews, *Effective Health Care* bulletins, *Effectiveness Matters*, the Database of Abstracts of Reviews of Effectiveness (see the Cochrane Library), the HTA Database (containing abstracts produced by the International Network of Agencies for Health Technology Assessment) and the NHS National Economic Evaluation Database (NEED).	NHS CRD University of York Heslington, York YO1 5DD Tel: 01904 433648 Fax: 01904 433661 E-mail: revdis@york.ac.uk http://www.york.ac.uk/inst.crd/info.htm *Effective Health Care* bulletins and *Effectiveness Matters* available from: FT Healthcare, Maple House 149 Tottenham Court Road London W1P 9LL Tel: 0171 896 2409 Fax: 0171 896 2213
NHS R & D Health Technology Assessments Programme	Health Technology Assessment is the largest single programme of work within the NHS Research and Development Programme. 'Health technology' covers all interventions including the use of devices, equipment, drugs, procedures and care across the whole spectrum of medical, nursing and health practices. The programme aims to address the questions of purchasers, providers and users of health services on the effectiveness and cost-effectiveness of interventions.	Programme Manager's Office National Coordinating Centre for Health Technology Assessment Mailing 928, Boldrewood University of Southampton Highfield, Southampton SO16 7PX Tel: 01703 595586 Fax: 01703 595639 E-mail: hta@soton.ac.uk
HTA Database	A database maintained by the NHS CRD of UK and international Health Technology Assessments, including INAHTA (International Network of Agencies for Health Technology Assessment) abstracts.	From the NHS CRD, see above.
Development and Evaluation Committee reports, Wessex Institute	These reports are prepared as part of the Development and Evaluation Service funded by the R & D Directorate South and West. They are intended to provide rapid, accurate and usable information on health technology effectiveness to purchasers, clinicians, managers and researchers in the South and West.	Development and Evaluation Committee Wessex Institute Biomedical Sciences Building Bassett Crescent East Southampton SO16 7PX http://www.epi.bris.ac.uk/rd

Economic evaluations

Source	Remit of information source	Contact details
NHS Economic Evaluations Database (NEED)	Produced by the NHS CRD (see above).	Available from the NHS CRD (see above).

Information for patients

Source	Remit of information source	Contact details
Centre for Health Information Quality (CHiQ)	CHiQ is working to support the development of information for patients which is clearly communicated, evidence-based and involves the patients.	Centre for Health Information Quality Highcroft, Romsey Road Winchester SO22 5DH Tel: 01962 863511, ext. 200 Fax: 01962 849079/840454 E-mail: enquiries@centreforhiq. demon.co.uk http://www.centreforhiq.demon.co.uk

Outcomes

Source	Remit of information source	Contact details
UK Clearing House on Health Outcomes	The UK Clearing House on Health Outcomes was established in 1992 and is funded by the NHS Executive, Scottish Home and Health Department, Welsh Office and Northern Ireland Department of Health and Social Services. It was set up to provide information and advice to the UK NHS on outcome measures and outcome measurement. It maintains databases of outcomes activities and structured abstracts.	UK Clearing House on Health Outcomes Nuffield Institute for Health 71–75 Clarendon Road Leeds LS2 9PL Tel: 0113 233 3940 Fax: 0113 246 0899 E-mail: hsschho@leeds.ac.uk http://www.leeds.ac.uk/nuffield/ infoservices/UKCH/home.html

Evidence-based information for purchasers

Source	Remit of information source	Contact details
Trent Working Group on Acute Purchasing	The Trent Working Group on Acute Purchasing was set up to enable purchasers to share research knowledge about the effectiveness and cost-effectiveness of acute service interventions and determining collectively their purchasing policy. Produces guidance notes for purchasers.	Senior Information Officer Trent Institute for Health Services Research Regent Court 30 Regent Street Sheffield S1 4DA Tel: 0114 222 5420 Fax: 0114 272 4095 E-mail: scharrlib@sheffield.ac.uk http://www.shef.ac.uk/~tiwgap/

Evidence-based information for purchasers (continued)

Source	Remit of information source	Contact details
Scottish Health Purchasing Information Centre (SHPIC)	Remit is to analyse research evidence on the effectiveness of health service interventions, to assess the benefits and costs, and provide concise reports for purchasers, in non-technical language.	Programme Manager, SHPIC Summerfield House 2 Eday Road, Aberdeen AB15 6RE http://www.nhsconfed.net/shpic/doc01.htm
Evidence-based Purchasing, NHS Executive South and West	Evidence-based Purchasing is a bi-monthly digest of outputs from the NHS Executive R & D programme, intended to support evidence-based health care.	NHS Executive South and West Research and Development Directorate Canynge Hall, Whiteladies Road Clifton, Bristol BS8 2PR Tel: 0117 9287224 Fax: 0117 9287204 http://www.epi.bris.ac.uk/rd/publicat/ebpurch/index.htm
Health Evidence bulletins – Wales	Health Evidence bulletins – Wales are a new initiative in the field of health information since they act as signposts to the best current evidence across a broad range of evidence types and subject areas.	Protocol Enhancement Project Duthie Library UWCM, Cardiff CF4 4XN E-mail: weightmanal@cardiff.ac.uk http://www.uwcm.ac.uk/uwcm/lb/pep/index.html

Critically appraised research summaries

Source	Remit of information source	Contact details
Evidence-Based Medicine Evidence-Based Nursing Evidence-Based Mental Health	From the BMJ Publishing Group. These journals aim to keep the clinician up to date by using scientific criteria to select and abstract the most reliable and important clinically relevant papers from an expanded range of journals. (Evidence-Based Medicine is available, along with the ACP Journal Club (see below), on CD-ROM (called Best Evidence) in the UK from the BMJ Publishing Group.)	BMJ Publishing Group BMA House Tavistock Square London WC1H 9JP Tel: 0171 387 4499 http://www.bmjpg.com/
Evidence-Based Health Policy and Management	Provides managers with the best evidence available about the financing, organisation and delivery of health care. Published by Churchill Livingstone.	Subscriptions from: Journals Subscription Department Harcourt Brace and Company Ltd Foots Cray High Street Sidcup, Kent DA14 5HP Tel: 0181 300 3322 http://www.ihs.ox.ac.uk/ebhpm
Evidence-Based Practice POEMs (Patient-Oriented Evidence that Matters)	The journal Evidence-Based Practice is produced by the publishers of the Journal of Family Practice. It identifies studies which meet criteria for relevance to the patients and practice of primary care physicians and calls these POEMs – Patient-Oriented Evidence that Matters. Once they have identified a POEM they assess the validity of the research and publish a synopsis.	Orders: Tel: 01 800 451 3794 Fax: 01 203 406 4603 http://jfp.msu.edu/ebp.htm

Critically appraised research summaries (continued)

Source	Remit of information source	Contact details
ACP Journal Club, American College of Physicians	Published six times a year, *ACP Journal Club* takes a "best of the best" approach, providing succinct summaries and expert commentaries on internal medicine topics. Only those that meet explicit standards for high scientific merit for clinical practice are chosen for inclusion. Available, along with *Evidence-Based Medicine*, on CD-ROM (called *Best Evidence*) in the UK from the BMJ Publishing Group – see above.	American College of Physicians Independence Mall West Sixth Street at Race Philadelphia, PA 19106-1572 Tel:001 800 523 1546 Fax: 001 215 351 2644 E-mail: ebm@mail.acponline.org
Bandolier	*Bandolier* is produced monthly in Oxford for the NHS R & D Directorate. It contains bullet points (hence *Bandolier*) of evidence-based medicine.	Available from Oxford and Anglia NHS Region R & D: Tel: 01865 226132 Fax: 01865 226978
Therapeutics Initiative	The Therapeutics Initiative was been established in 1994 by the Department of Pharmacology and Therapeutics in cooperation with the Department of Family Practice at the University of British Columbia to provide physicians and pharmacists with up to date, evidence-based, practical information on rational drug therapy. The initiative is an independent organisation, which is at arm's length from government, pharmaceutical industry and other vested interest groups.	http://interchg.ubc.ca/jauca/
The National Preferred Medicines Centre Inc (PreMeC)	PreMeC is based in New Zealand and was founded "by GPs, for GPs" in 1991. Participation in PreMeC activities is entirely voluntary. It is a proactive, independent agency, free from ulterior motives or vested interests. It promotes best-practice, evidence-based prescribing.	PO Box 10–545 Level 3, 88 The Terrace Wellington, New Zealand Tel: 64 04 496 5960 Fax: 64 04 496 5961 E-mail: kerry@rnzcgp.org.nz
Aggressive Research Intelligence Facility (ARIF)	ARIF is a specialist unit based at the University of Birmingham, set up to help health care workers access and interpret research evidence in response to particular problems.	ARIF 27 Highfield Road Edgbaston Birmingham B15 3DP Tel/fax: 0121 455 6852 E-mail: c.j.hyde@bham.ac.uk http://www.hsrc.org.uk/links/arif/arifhome.htm
Critically Appraised Topics (CAT) Bank	The CAT Bank is a storage and retrieval facility for a collection of CATs (critically appraised topics) provided by the Centre for Evidence-Based Medicine, Oxford. The Centre for Evidence-Based Mental Health is currently developing a CAT Bank specific to mental health (see listing under Centre for Evidence-Based Mental Health).	Centre Coordinator NHS R & D Centre for Evidence-Based Medicine Nuffield Department of Clinical Medicine, University of Oxford Level 5, John Radcliffe Hospital Headington, Oxford OX3 9DU Tel: 01865 221321 Fax: 01865 222901 E-mail: oliveg@cebm.jr2.ox.ac.uk http://cebm.jr2.ox.ac.uk/docs/catbank.html

Other

Source	Remit of information source	Contact details
Professional bodies relevant to the EBB topic area	Royal College of Physicians' Research Unit reports and *Linker* – the newsletter of the National R & D Network in the Health Care of Older People.	Research Unit Royal College of Physicians 11 St Andrews Place London NW1 4LE Tel: 0171 935 2711 Fax: 0171 487 3988 E-mail: linker@rcplondon.ac.uk
	American Association on Mental Retardation	American Association on Mental Retardation Alzheimer's Disease Workgroup 444 North Capitol Street, NW Suite 846 Washington DC
	National Center for Cost Containment	National Center for Cost Containment Department of Veterans Affairs 5000 West National Avenue Milwaukee, WI 53295, USA
Voluntary sector organisations relevant to the EBB topic area	Alzheimer's Disease Society	Alzheimer's Disease Society Gordon House 10 Greencoat Place London SW1P 1PH
A list of additional voluntary sector organisations, and patient and carer support groups is available from the RCPsych Research Unit (see above)	The Alzheimer Society of Canada	Alzheimer Society of Canada 1320 Yonge Street Suite 201 Toronto, ON M4T 1X2 Canada
Department of Health	Circulars on the Internet (COIN) database allows searching of DOH reports and papers.	http://tap.ccta.gov.uk/doh/coin.nsf
Joseph Rowntree Foundation	The Joseph Rowntree Foundation (JRF) supports a programme of research and development in the fields of housing, social care and social policy. JRF research findings and reports can be searched by topic on the website.	Joseph Rowntree Foundation The Homestead 40 Water End York YO3 6LP Tel: 01904 629241 Fax: 01904 620072 www: http://www.jrf.org.uk/

Feedback form

We hope that you have found this evidence-base briefing (EBB) useful and we would very much appreciate your feedback. Your comments will be incorporated, where possible, into future editions of this publication.

(1)   Have you found this EBB useful? 5 Yes 5 No

If yes, please describe briefly how the EBB has been used in practice.

. . . .
. . . .
. . . .
. . . .

(2)   Are there sources of evidence that you think ought to have been included in this EBB?
Please list full references where possible.

. . . .
. . . .
. . . .
. . . .

(3)   Do you have suggestions for topics areas in which you would like to see future EBBs developed?

. . . .
. . . .
. . . .

(4)   Do you have any general suggestions about this EBB which would improve its usefulness?

. . . .
. . . .
. . . .

(5)   What is your profession?

(6)   How many people in your organisation have access to this EBB?

If you have any further comments, please continue overleaf.

Thank you for taking the time to complete this form. Your comments will be considered carefully.

Please photocopy and return to:

Claire Palmer, Royal College of Psychiatrists' Research Unit, FREEPOST – LON602, 11 Grosvenor Crescent, London, SW1X 7YS